My Brave Face

A Memoir of Love and Courage Through The Life Of My Son

Heather Simpson

My Brave Face: A Memoir of Love and Courage Through The Life Of My Son

First published in Australia 2021 by Heather Simpson

ISBN 978-0-6452521-0-1

Disclaimer

All the information, techniques, skills and concepts contained within this publication are of the nature of general comment only and are not in any way recommended as individual advice. The intent is to offer a variety of information to provide a wider range of choices now and in the future, recognising that we all have widely diverse circumstances and viewpoints. Should any reader choose to make use of the information herein, this is their decision, and the author and publisher/s do not assume any responsibilities whatsoever under any conditions or circumstances. The author does not take responsibility for the business, financial, personal or other success, results or fulfilment upon the readers' decision to use this information. It is recommended that the reader obtain their own independent advice.

This book is dedicated to Stephen.

There is no higher honour than the privilege of being your mother.
My memories of you are the treasure of my life, precious beyond compare.

Table of Contents

Introduction

My name is Heather Simpson. I was born in Fremantle, Western Australia, on May 22, 1940.

I would like you to come on a journey with me, my husband Ray and our son Stephen, to whom this book is dedicated. It will be a journey that crosses the globe, a mix of pleasure, pain, humour, music and never-ending love.

This is the true story of how we dealt with the painful bone disease Osteogenesis Imperfecta (OI), or brittle bones, as a family, by always keeping a positive attitude and never ever giving up.

OI sufferers have been reported to range between 2.35 to 4.7 in 100,000 worldwide with no preference for race or gender. It can express itself in different forms of severity from mild to severe. In some cases, this inherited bone fragility can cause catastrophic, lifelong disability with enormous ramifications for both the long-suffering individual and their family.

'Brittle bones' is the common name for the disease. Because I was born with a mild form of this condition, I have, over the years, undertaken a rigorous research journey to understand this disease and how to live with it.

When I was diagnosed as a young girl, even the doctors knew little about this condition. It is a collagen disorder that affects the matrix of the bone. Collagen comes from a Greek word meaning 'glue'. In OI, the collagen decreases in both quantity and quality. This means that bones can go soft like plasticine and bend into odd shapes, yet can be easily broken and shatter like glass with the least amount of provocation.

In an otherwise healthy body, the skeleton of the bone is completely renewed and replaced with new bone every five to ten years. In OI sufferers, the old bone is not completely renewed, and the absence of glue or collagen leaves the bones old, crumbling, soft or brittle. OI cannot be cured by simply taking calcium, as is commonly perceived, because the bone does not absorb the calcium, similar to oil on water.

We were young, Ray and I, when we had Stephen. The three of us grew up together. Having this condition resulted in a myriad of challenges. However, the biggest challenge was not from the disease itself, but from people's attitudes – self-absorbed doctors and bureaucracies making a combination for getting nowhere fast.

I hope that telling my story and sharing my deepest thoughts and feelings about us and our son Stephen, will help other sufferers struggling with physical or personal hardships. His endurance with his pain, and my never-ending hope for the future, will tug at your heart strings. The concepts of this story may be applied to anyone living with a disability. If this book gets just one person to reconsider how they treat people with a disability, then all the time, tears and effort it took me to write it will be worth it. Will that person be you?

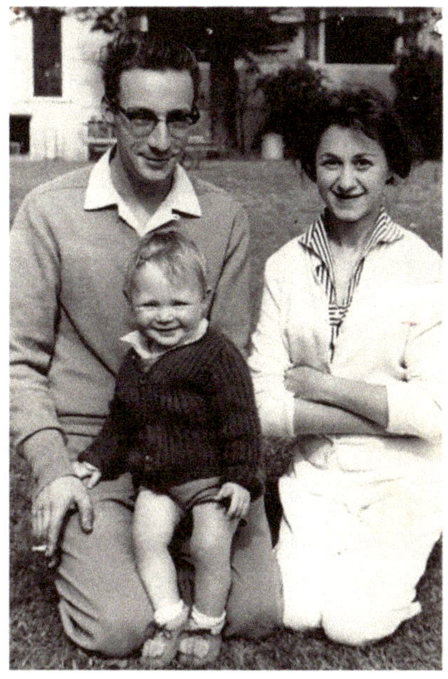

Ray, me and Stevie at 16 months

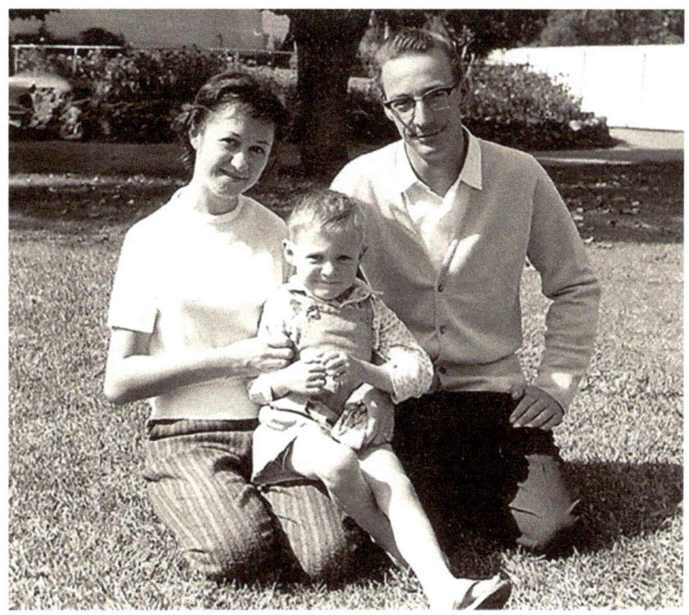

Ray, me and Stevie at 3 years

PART 1: THE EARLY YEARS

MY CHILDHOOD AND STEPHEN AGE 0–7

1

The Start of Our Long and Winding Road

This story begins with me, with what happened to me long before my son arrived.

I was born in 1940 with a less severe form of OI than what my son Stephen would eventually be diagnosed with. I was a very thin and frail child dealing with the terrible pain of repeatedly breaking bones causing long hospitalisations. Although the disease is usually inherited through genetics, I was just unlucky and experienced what the doctors called a 'spontaneous mutation'.

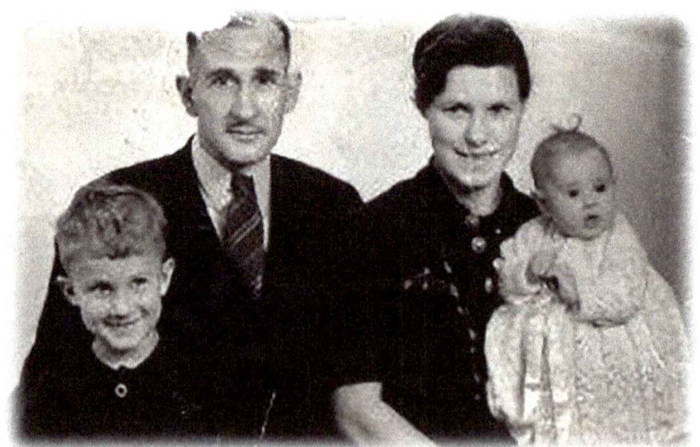

My brother Tommy, my parents and me in 1940

My mother told me that my first misfortune happened in 1942 when I was aged two. My overweight cousin jumped from a wall and landed on top of me, breaking my leg. I can vaguely remember being in bed with a thick plaster on, but I was not held back for long. I grew stronger after healing from my first fracture.

At the back of our big house were horse stables. On this day, there was a horse bucking wildly in the corral. As a two-year-old toddler who had just recovered from her first fracture, I came out our back door and just walked up to the horse in the corral. The horse stopped bucking and looked down at me snorting, as I placed my two little hands on its knees. It shook and trembled but did not hurt me. Everyone was screaming.

"Look at Heather, my God, she is going to get killed! The horse will kill her! Get her out! Get her out!"

The horse, not moving a muscle, gazed quietly down at me. At that moment I had no fear. Then to everyone's relief, I just turned around and casually toddled out of the corral, unfazed. Given my dad was a gifted horseman, it appeared I had inherited his love and connection with horses, and I developed a lifelong love for the 'horse'.

My brother, Tommy, remembers we later lived in another house in Alexander Street in East Fremantle in Western Australia. It was constructed with jarrah wood and had a big veranda all around. One day, my brother aged 9 and I aged 5 were sitting on the veranda when we felt very hungry. My mother was in bed sleeping. Tommy decided to make us a sandwich. He crushed up some garden snails, removing all the shells. He pulled the middle out from a loaf of bread and folded it over the snails. As we ate, we both thought it was delicious.

A nasty teacher once broke my arm by hitting it with a thick ruler. She also whacked the back of my legs for sneezing too loudly, crazily proclaiming that I had sneezed on purpose. To this day, I stifle my sneeze with little sound due to the trauma this incident caused me. My legs, that time, held up and did not break – they were just bruised black and blue. Teachers were permitted to mete out 'discipline' how they saw fit in those days.

I recall long periods being fracture-free when I could play normal childhood games. I would skip rope for hours and walk three miles to school, which no doubt strengthened my bones temporarily. However, these long absences of pain would eventually be interrupted when I broke collar bones, ribs, and even my legs one after the other. It was a common event for me to fracture a leg, and just when it had mended, the same leg or the other leg would break again. I suppose I was lucky to usually have one mended leg, and so could get around on crutches. I soon learned that crutches were extremely dangerous. They could slip from under your arms if you used them on a slippery surface, and I would then hear the resounding 'crack' of my weight putting sudden unexpected pressure on an unsuspecting limb, breaking the leg.

I was in and out of hospital with various mishaps. Hospitals then were very strictly regimented. The Head Sister would tour the wards and inspect every bed periodically for wrinkles, as if she had nothing better to do. Patients had to be tucked in tightly and uncomfortably with not a crease showing in the sheets; otherwise, the Head Sister would chastise the nurses severely. She was a 'control freak', and the nurses were always afraid of her. So much for the hospital supposedly being a place of caring for patients.

When I was six years old, my mother and I went to Petersham, a suburb in Sydney NSW to visit her mother. I broke my collarbone by tripping over the backdoor steps. My mother was very mad and upset with me, as if I had broken the bone deliberately. She was already in a state of despair and could not handle more bad news. Thereafter, I was always afraid about her finding out I had broken a bone, and on these occasions, when in the hospital, I would beg for the nurses not to tell my mother. I wanted to protect her from further grief. I now see they had to tell her, as I would be missing from the family home.

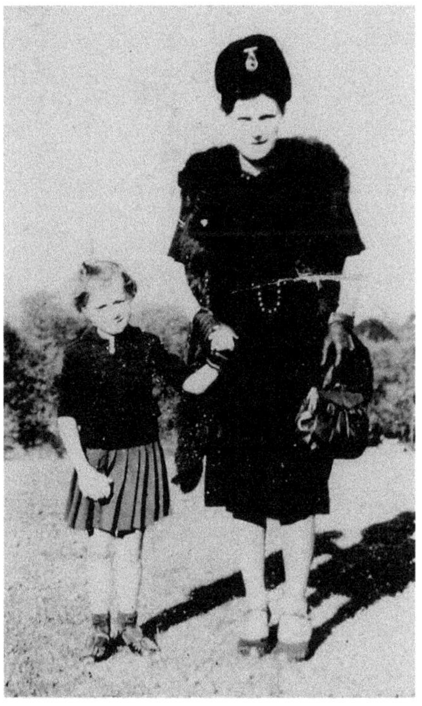

My mother and me in Sydney, 1946

In 1948 when I was eight, my father, an Englishman aged 48 died from tuberculosis. According to my mother, he contracted the lung disease while serving for eight years in the British Army in India. One day I came home from school and my mother was in our shoe repair shop, sitting on the couch and crying. I asked Tommy what was wrong with Mummy. This is how he tried to explain to me what had happened:

"You know that song we listen to That Little Kid Sister of Mine?"

I nodded. The song describes a new star that was needed in heaven, but they could not find a bright-enough light to shine. God decided the little kid-sister was meant to be the new star, so He sent for 'that little kid sister' to be the new star up yonder.

Tommy described how the girl in the song went to heaven and then told me, "Well, that's where Dad has gone." I started laughing and thought, "Gee, something exciting has happened for once in the family and Dad is in heaven. This is just great!"

As I was only a child, I had no real concept of death, until it hit me whilst on a holiday. Family rallied around us, and we went to stay with my mother's aunt for three weeks as my mother was grieving and in shock and needed support. During that stay, I once woke up in the middle of the night, crying as I realised I wasn't going to see Daddy anymore. It had only just occurred to me that what had happened was final.

My mother rushed in and asked, "What is the matter?"

"I want my daddy, I won't see my daddy anymore," I cried out over and over.

Subsequently, everyone else started crying too.

My father's brothers being of the Catholic faith were always against my parents marrying in The Church of England in Fremantle, as my mother was Scottish and not a Catholic. My mother not being a Catholic was the first of many things that provoked them to disapprove of her. Further, when I was seven, my father had taken me on his bicycle to make my First Holy Communion in the Catholic Church, but my mother had run alongside and pulled me off the bike, screaming, "You are not taking her!" This further divided the family.

Later at my father's funeral, there was a disgusting commotion due to the long-standing bitterness over differences of faith. As my father was being lowered into the Protestant Soldiers' Section of the cemetery, my father's brothers threw rosary beads onto his coffin. This enraged my mother so much that she tried to jump into the grave to throw the beads out, but her sisters pulled her back. This was just another distressing incident, taking its toll on my mother.

Soon after, I became terribly ill with peritonitis and almost died. A pastor was called to give me last rites and my mother kept crying. I remember the doctor cutting my ankle to insert a tube to give me a blood transfusion, which ultimately saved my life. My mother and brother each were given a bed nearby and stayed round the clock at the hospital. During fits of delirium, I begged my mother to get me a horse to come home to. She and Tommy promised they had bought a horse and it was in the back yard waiting for me to come home. That acted as a trigger for my recovery, for I could not wait to see my horse.

When I was well enough and went home, I was distraught to find there was no horse. Tommy, who had pushed all the grass down by the back fence, said the horse had run away. I disbelieved him but he came back and said, "See where the horse has eaten all the grass?" I was dejected to say the least and I suspected the whole thing had been a big fat lie to quickly get me well.

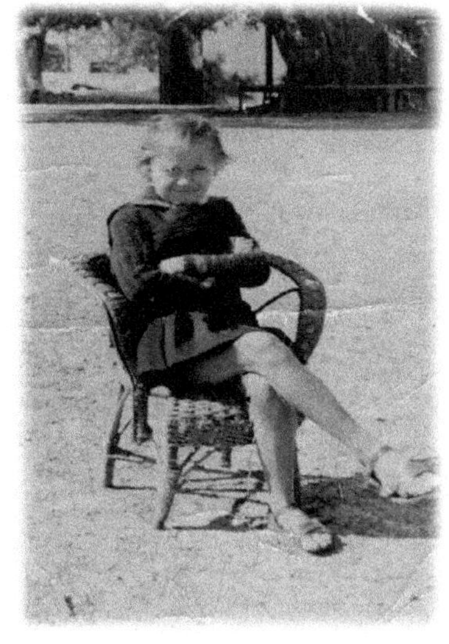

After recovery from peritonitis, 1948

I may not have got the horse I longed for, but I did get a little black-and-white Fox Terrier, named Skippy. He was a great little companion. Sadly, in just a few months, he was hit by a car. I was only eight and heartbroken when Skippy died in my arms. Then I would bring home stray cats, begging my mother to let me keep them. I acquired both nits and ringworms during this time and had to have my head shaved.

I was very weak after the bout of peritonitis, so Tommy built a billycart with wheels and pushed me everywhere in it. Those were very rough rides, stumbling over rocks and tram lines, and banging into lamp posts, gutters and anything in the way. One day we were going to our shoe repair shop in Adelaide Street, Fremantle, when a wheel came off the billycart while crossing the tram line. We always carried a hammer in case the cart fell to pieces. Before the tram came, Tommy quickly hammered in the nail to connect the wheel back to the cart. Despite my brittle bones, I miraculously survived this rough transportation treatment. It was so much fun and one of the happiest memories of my childhood.

As I grew stronger and free of plaster casts for a while, the circus came to a recreation park not far from our house in High Street, Fremantle. To me, a circus meant horses. I ran out to the bus stop in my excitement, where a man in a dark coat was also standing. I wondered what the time was and if I would have time to see the horses before I went shopping for dinner. I went up to the man and asked him the time. He said that he would show me the time, and the next thing I remember is following him – he may have led me by the hand. I have banished from my memory the exact scene of what followed. He took me to the toilets at the back of the Four-Square Park. He showed me his member, which frightened me, and I ran out from the toilet all the way to where the horses were in the circus.

At the circus, I found several ponies standing together. Nothing has ever deterred me from patting horses on their noses, which are so amazingly soft to touch. One of the kids there pointed to a nice little horse and said, "Pat that one!" When I reached out to pat the horse, it suddenly laid its ears back and bit me on the chest. I got home from the circus in tears. But my mother gave me the biggest hiding with a belt, yelling, "I told you never to talk to strangers, didn't I?" over and over with each whack from the belt. It just so happened that a woman had seen the paedophile take me to the toilet and told my mother.

I was taken to a doctor for examination that thankfully revealed I was not interfered with. Consequently, a court case developed over the whole episode, and it ended with the judge giving me a handful of coins indicating that I had won the case against that disgusting man.

I knew well the isolation of being a sick child. In addition to physical pain, I experienced emotional pain with the loss of my father. The loss took a bodily and mental toll on my mother too, who became severely depressed and would spend most of her time lying in bed. I felt like I was a burden to her.

She was trying to maintain the shoe repair business which my father had started in the 1930s after returning from serving in the British Army in India. To help with household expenses, my brother Tommy took on a little job selling afternoon newspapers. He then left school at 14 years of age to learn the shoe repair trade from a family friend in the same business. After training there, he would go into our shop to work with mother until closing time.

Because my mother and brother were trying to keep everything together, I had to help after school by learning to cook. In between my hospitalisations and episodes of sickness, life was hard for all of us. I had to stand and walk on two painful weak legs to get things done. I would go to the food shops after school to get meat and vegetables to cook our evening meal. To their amusement and my embarrassment, I would hear the check-out girls say, "Here comes little mother."

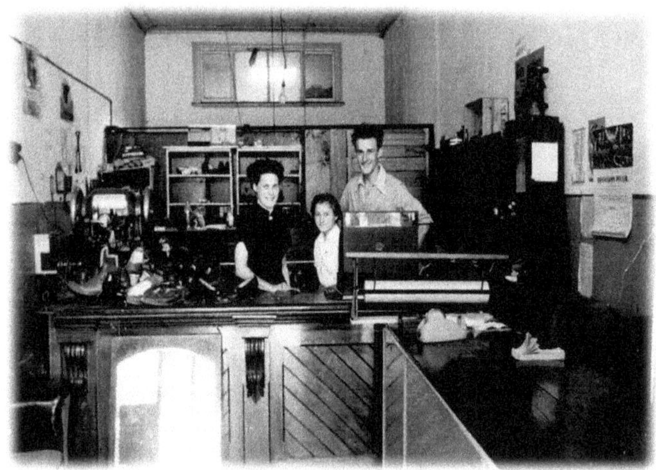

Me with my mother and brother in 1953

One morning, seeing there was not enough milk, my mother told me to go get some. I got on my scooter and raced to the shop. I was in such a hurry that I lost my balance and fell, breaking my leg. My mother would be so distraught with every break I had that she would invariably spend more and more time in bed.

Business at the shoe repair shop was slow. We had to move out of our rented house to live behind our shoe repair shop. Because we had sheets of leather for mending shoes, the place was overrun with rats. I would wake up most nights 'smelling a rat' as they had a distinct foul odour, and often find one scurrying over me where I slept on the couch. I trembled under the covers. We survived like this for five years until my mother sold the business and built a new house.

During this time, my father's brothers tried to get the government welfare agency to put us into a 'good Catholic home'. My mother fought tooth and nail to keep us together.

Having lost my father due to war causes, I was a 'legacy ward' and received free medical treatment in Hollywood Hospital, a repatriation hospital for ex-soldiers' and deceased soldiers' families. When I was in there, I was worried I would never leave, as I had heard many people say that once you went in there, you would never get out alive.

In 1953, at the age of thirteen, I was admitted to Hollywood Hospital for several months for an assessment of my condition. While there one day, my femur (thigh bone) cracked. The sickening sound of it surged through my body like lightning. Some weeks later, turning over, the other femur cracked, so then I had two legs in traction. It was a very lonely time. My mother was always sick and could seldom visit me in hospital, since it entailed catching two buses and a long walk. Having a car was a luxury in those days that few could afford.

On Sundays, which was visiting day, I would hide under the sheet when all the visitors came because I felt embarrassed for not having any visitors. My mother tried her best by writing beautiful letters, which I have kept to this day. I would read them over and over and be consoled by her calling me her 'own darling little lassie'. I knew that she felt sorry for me and loved me.

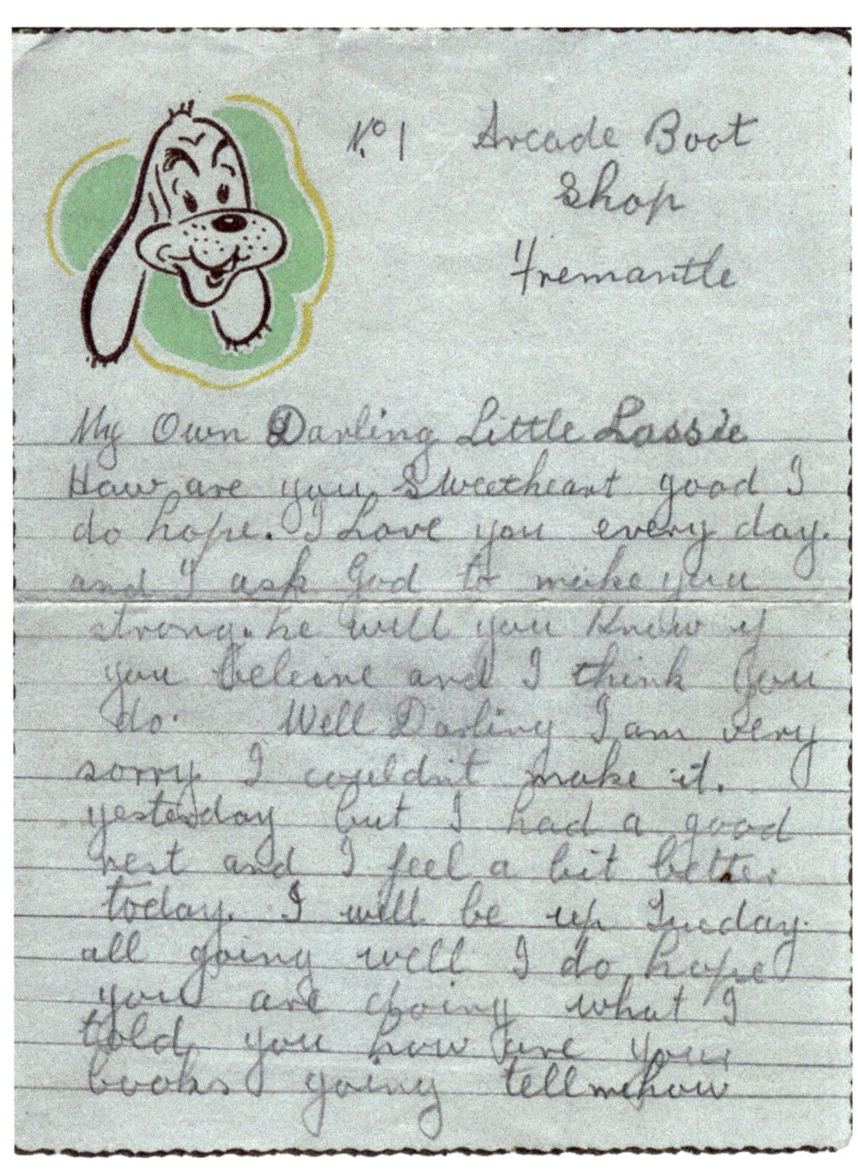

No 1 Arcade Boot
Shop
Fremantle

My Own Darling Little Lassie
How are you Sweetheart good I
do hope. I Love you every day.
and I ask God to make you
strong. he will you know if
you beleive and I think you
do. Well Darling I am very
sorry I couldn't make it.
yesterday but I had a good
rest and I feel a bit better
today. I will be up Tuesday
all going well I do hope
you are doing what I
told you how are your
books going tell me how

2

much you have read when I come
up & do keep yourself bright
& happy & see Beauty in
every thing & then you
will be happy now don't
you think it is a lot of
fun watching all the Ladies
you want to write down
every day what you see
funny & read it to me
when I come up to see
you & we can have a
real good Laugh together
now don't you think that
would be fun now how
about starting now I am
sure you can see something
right now to write about,
well Darling [illegible] Your Loving Mummy x x x x x xx x

Treasured letter from my mother I have kept since I was 13 years old

However, there was one special visitor I should mention. In February 1954, Queen Elizabeth of England came to Perth and made a visit to Hollywood Hospital, where I was again a patient. It was arranged that I present her with a bouquet from my wheelchair. I remember how beautiful and fair she looked. Even today, I look back at it with a smile and see how special it was to meet The Queen of England.

2

More Pain Before Gain

At 14 years of age, I enrolled in my first year of high school. My legs were weak following my long stay at the hospital, and could hardly bear my weight even with the aid of crutches. My brother Tommy at that time was working in our shoe repair shop close by. Every day he would transport me to and from school on his bicycle. I had not been there long when a fellow student, who was carrying me down some stairs, tripped and dropped me. My leg broke again. Tommy came to get me and back I went into hospital.

After months of rehabilitation, doctors told me that the next time I broke my legs they would do surgery to straighten the bones. I asked, "Why can't you just do it before I break my leg to save going through that pain of the break again?" My tibia bones (shin bones) had begun to badly bend forward from the repeated breaks, a common occurrence with this disease. The doctors eventually decided it was time to operate to straighten my legs. The procedure consisted of breaking the tibias in multiple places in both legs, rotating the sections to reduce the curve and resetting the tibias. The subsequent pain was incredibly intense and the only analgesia available was aspirin, which did little to ease the pain.

Soon after surgery, I was forced to stand and walk with blood-stained casts on each leg. With each step, I had tears streaming down my face as a sickening wave of pain surged through me. Still, I was happy because my legs looked straight.

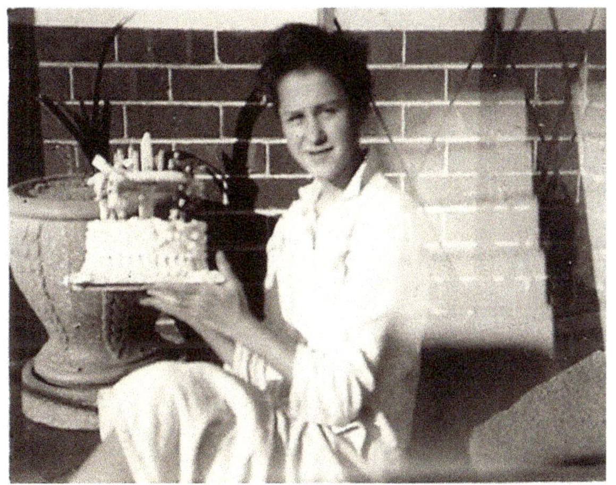

Recovering on my fourteenth birthday, 1954

I had a long recovery period in bed at home. During this time, I made myself busy by knitting, crocheting, reading and listening to radio serials Portia Faces Life and Blue Hills broadcast every day from 1:00 PM. I had marvellous company with me all day on my bed with my little black cat Moogy-Meow. I often spent many hours drawing horses.

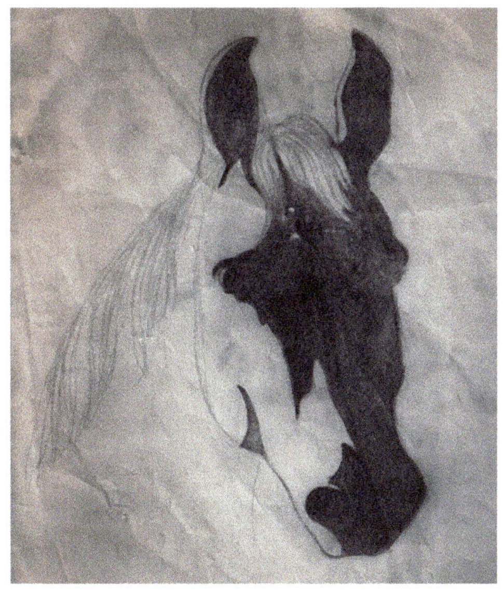

A drawing I did in 1954

I had no doubt inherited my love for horses from my father, who had been a mounted Trooper with the British Army in India. My father had been very skilled with his hands. He had made sandals every summer for me and my brother. He also made all sorts of cowboy paraphernalia. His idol was movie actor Tom Mix who made westerns from 1910 to 1940. My father could match the cowboy skills of the Tom Mix movies. His horse looked like Tom Mix's horse with a white blaze on the face and two white back legs. He had also learned knife throwing, trick riding, whip cracking, lassoing and rope tricks.

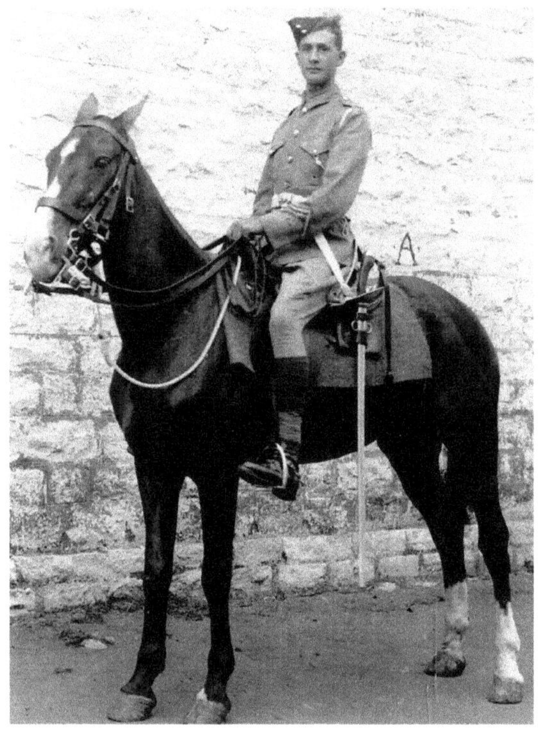

My father as a Trooper in the British Army in India, 1919

In the years before World War II, there was a rodeo every Friday night in Fremantle. My father would have my mother stand against

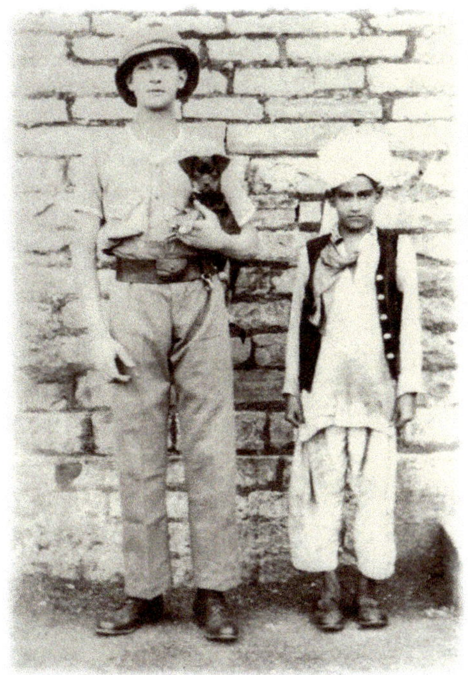

My Father in the British Army in India, 1919

a wooden door, and he would throw knives all around her like a Kung Fu master. He was also proficient with a whip, and Tommy and I would help him practise. We would hold the ends of a rolled-up newspaper in our mouth and our father would split it in two by cracking the whip. We thought it was fun and were never afraid. We loved the cracking sound the whip made. He could do all types of

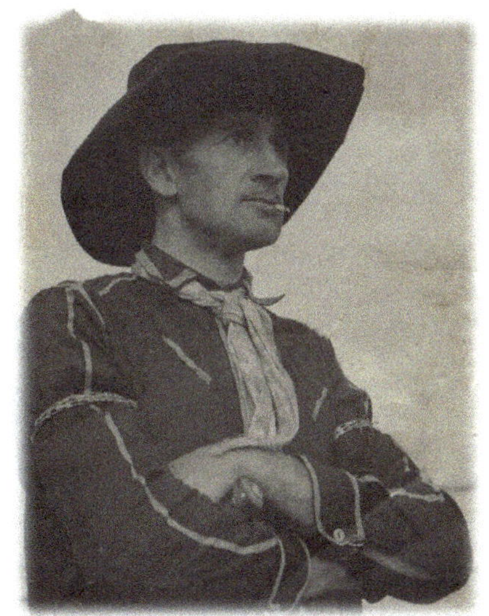

My father, the cowboy in Fremantle, 1939

tricks at the rodeo, jumping in and out of spinning ropes. He was a real cowboy.

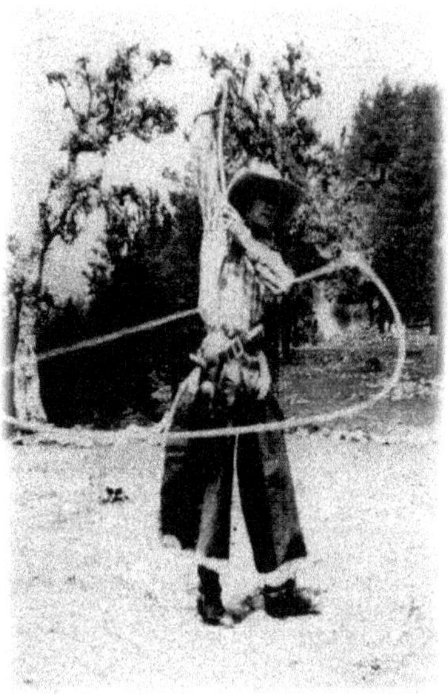

My father, aged 22, doing rope tricks in Canada

After the operations, my legs were so weak that they quickly bent again under the strain of supporting my body, despite my being underweight. My bones were just too soft. I was devastated.

I spent my early teens until I was 15 recuperating and being careful not to have any more setbacks. After a year of convalescing, I started to think about what I could do for a future career. I had to get a job to help pay for household expenses. In my heart I wanted to be a nurse, but I knew that the physical demands of nursing did not make it a viable career choice due to my disability.

The only job I could find at that time was at a department store which naturally involved a lot of standing. The pain in my legs from standing all day was indescribable. I dreaded getting on the bus to go home. I was afraid to sit down because when I got up again, the pain surging through my legs would be so intense that I could hardly breathe. I would grip the bus post tightly, hoping the pain would stop and praying I would not collapse.

I decided to attend a commercial college and study stenography for two years. In order to get a job, I knew I had to be better than anyone else, and so I practised typing page after page to improve my speed and accuracy. I was very focussed on achieving good results. Conscious of my legs, I put my head down and studied hard. Soon I was able to accurately type 120 words per minute and write 100 words per minute in shorthand. Even to this day, it is still the beautiful people who get the jobs. Therefore, back then as a 17-year-old, I wore my skirts long to hide my legs. Potential employers would balk at hiring a person with distorted legs or any disability in case of compensation claims on the job.

As fate would have it, my life was about to change. In 1957 at the age of 17, I met my 'knight in shining armour' and fell in love. I was walking down the street with a girlfriend when we spotted a young man running across the road towards us. My friend knew him as they worked at the same steel foundry. She introduced me to Raymond Simpson. Later that day, Ray sourced my phone number and called me, asking me if I would like to go to his friend's wedding that evening. I told him I couldn't go as it had been raining and all my freshly washed clothes were wet, leaving me with no dry clothes to wear. He would not accept this as an excuse.

Consequently, I ironed dry an outfit and went off to meet Ray. Thinking about my legs again, which now had a slight curve due to the nature of the disease, I was very hesitant to go. I was afraid that if he noticed them, he would lose interest in me. I had previously had a few boyfriends who never called me again after they had seen the state of my legs. I was very crushed by this, and it had damaged my self-esteem. It made me want to hide away from men. A teenager has a fragile sense of self at best.

I used to cry to my mother, “Everyone stares at my legs. I hate my legs!”

My mother was saddened by this and tried her best to reassure me that I would someday meet someone who would love me the way I was.

Shortly after I met Ray, I decided to test him one evening. Knowing he had not noticed my legs yet, I said slowly:

“I want to tell you something. I have a bent leg.”

“So what?” he replied.

I was surprised he had taken it so well. I continued, “Well, the other one is bent too.”

He sighed and said, “I love you for who you are, whether your legs be bent or straight.”

I was overjoyed and felt incredibly special that he accepted me for myself and did not care about my misshapen legs. I loved him for that. I recalled my mother’s words that I would someday meet someone who would love me the way I was.

Ray was gifted at writing poetry, and he would often send me flowers with verses he had composed. One particular verse I remember well.

Heather, let me tell you true,
I find I am in love with you.
You fill me with intense delight.
I long to stay with you all night,
Begging you with fervent pleas,
And even sinking to my knees
That you may kiss me once again,
In your embrace long to remain.

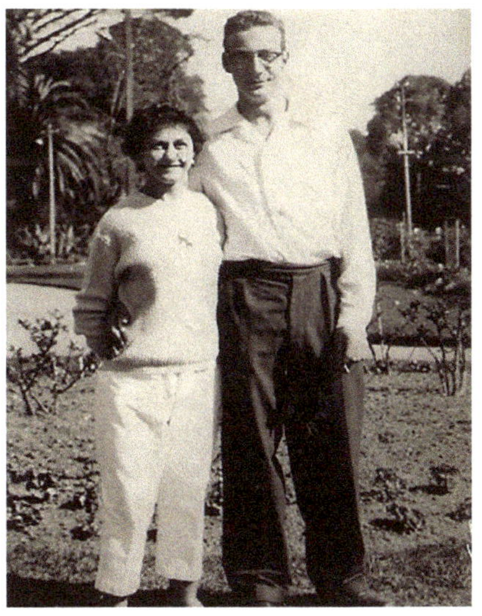

With Ray in Kings Park, 1957

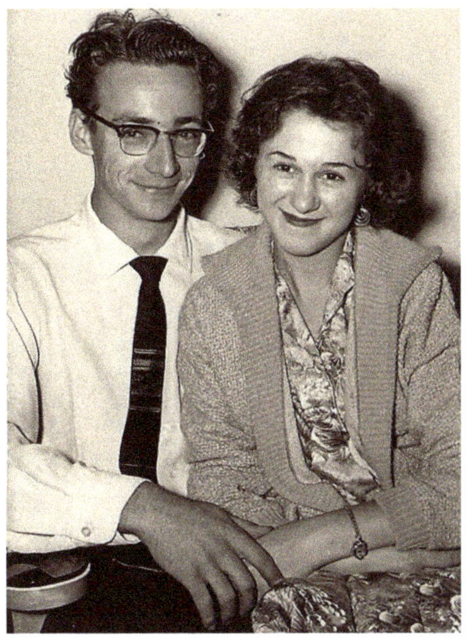

After our engagement, 1959

While courting, we would go to the pub for drinks with Ray's grandfather, Jim, and his wife, Ivy. It was all very 'respectable'. The pubs closed at 9:00 PM. I would sip on lemonade and Ray would drink a couple of beers. One night, while Ray was trying to get a taxi for me to go home, we started strolling in that direction. A taxi never showed, so we walked the whole way. Eventually, Ray and I got to my home around 1:00 AM. I very quietly opened the door, and was met by the 'thump-thump-thump' of my mother's angry footsteps charging down the passageway. Ray immediately jumped behind the front door.

"What are you doing coming home at this hour?" she screamed at me. It had previously been agreed I would be home by midnight. "He has no respect for you, coming home at this hour."

Just then she noticed Ray standing behind the door. Suddenly, her voice changed from a screaming banshee's to a friendly tone. "Oh, hello Ray," she said, and then pointed at me. "It's all her fault. I know what she's like."

Ray replied, "It's alright. After the pub closed, we went to my grandfather's house for a cup of tea. Had to walk home since we couldn't find a taxi."

"Well, that's alright then," she said calmly.

Other times when Ray came to visit, I would make him snacks and we would talk, and after a while he would say goodnight to my mother and me. Then he would go around to my bedroom window and climb in and get under my bed. My mother would sometimes come into my room and talk for two hours or more. During this time, I would be terrified that Ray would sneeze or cough and consequently be discovered. Now I think and laugh about it, because I am sure she knew Ray was under the bed. Mothers have an instinctive way of knowing what their children are up to, while we like to think we are getting away with our devious deeds. Sometimes, at 6:00 AM, Ray would get a lift home with the milkman who would ask Ray if he had been tomcatting around.

This whirlwind courtship of late nights took a toll on me. I found myself falling asleep at my desk often at my job as a stenographer. I would go to my boss and ask to go home, complaining of a headache. But he simply told me to lie down on my desk instead. So I would have a nap for two hours, and then get up and continue working. My boss thought the headaches were the stress of too much work, but I was just dead tired. This is a universal experience; when people fall in love, they want to spend every minute with that special person, and the common sense of getting a good night's sleep flies out the window.

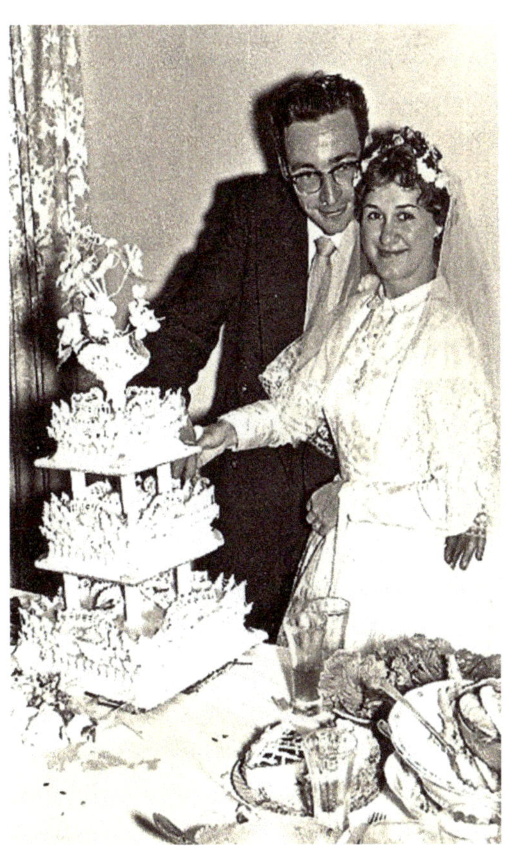

Our wedding day, October 1959

One day we were playfully pushing each other on a swing seat. Ray, not meaning to, pushed me too hard, and I fell onto the floor and broke my collarbone. Ray was shocked and could not believe what had happened. It was his first realization that my bones were delicate.

After two years of an exciting courtship, we got

married. I was happy at the thought of a new life with Ray, and with our baby on the way.

We lived with my mother for a few months, then moved to a rental house in South Fremantle.

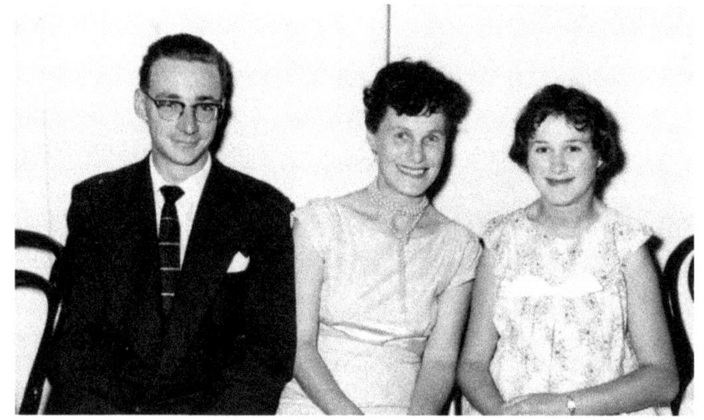

Ray, my mother, and me pregnant with Stephen

Stephen Alan Simpson was born on April 26, 1960, by caesarean section. The doctors had explained that there was a fifty percent chance that the baby would inherit my bone disease, so it would be safer to have a caesarean birth to prevent breaking his bones while being born. Pre-birth, there was no way of telling conclusively if he had brittle bones. Amniocentesis testing had not been perfected then.

At birth, Stephen was a perfectly formed baby. When I looked at him in my arms for the first time, I could not believe how beautiful this little boy looked. I was deliriously happy. Unfortunately, my happiness was short lived.

After five days, although Stephen was kicking his legs and waving his arms like any normal baby, the doctors suspected Stephen had inherited my brittle bone genes. The doctor explained to me that a significant diagnostic sign of the condition is the white part of the eye having a blue tinge, known as 'blue sclera'. And yes, indeed; Stephen's sclera was tinged with blue.

In those days, doctors were considered to be Gods. We eagerly hung on to everything they said and constantly sought any glimmer of hope or positive news.

In the back of my mind, I believed the doctors were wrong. My beautiful little boy looked so perfect, weighing in at 6lb 3oz, which was a good result for a petite woman like me who was only 152.4 centimetres tall.

Stephen had normal progress as a baby; he began playing at three months and learned sitting at six months. I would play peekaboo, suddenly appearing from behind a couch, and he would laugh heartily. The sound of a baby laughing is the sweetest sound in the world. It was pure joy.

My mother taught me a song that she used to sing to my brother when he was a baby:

Sweetest little fellow, everybody knows,
Don't know what to call him but he's mighty like a rose!
Looking at his mummy with eyes so shiny blue,
Makes you feel that heaven is coming close to you …

These are some of my treasured and happiest memories. However, I recall how one day Stephen, aged just two months, broke his ribs through crying. I was rocking him back and forth trying to soothe him when I heard a dull clicking sound coming from somewhere inside him. I asked Ray to hold him and rock him gently, and Ray could also hear the clicking sound. We rushed our baby to the hospital. After X-rays of his chest, the doctors informed us that Stephen had eight broken ribs. They gave me his bonnet and booties, saying that they would have to keep him in the hospital for a while. I looked down at his tiny bonnet and booties and felt my heart shattering to pieces.

After this incident, Stephen cried every day and night for four and half months. I was exhausted. When Stephen finally fell asleep for short periods, I would hurry around desperately trying to cook, clean, wash diapers (or 'nappies' as we called them in those days) and catch up on everything needing attention. I felt enormous distress, struggling day to day with the demands of caring for my family. Ray was apprehensive but always looked on the bright side and trusted the doctors' opinions.

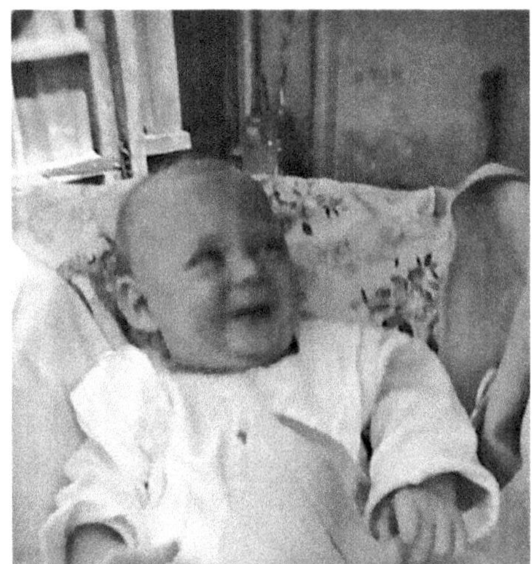

Stephen at 5 months

One night, as Ray lifted Stephen out of his bath, he began crying more than usual. We had come to assume at this point that every time he cried it meant a broken bone. We took him to the hospital. When we told the doctors that Stephen could have broken his ribs again, they implied that Ray had broken the baby's ribs. We had to explain that Stephen had a condition that meant he could cough and break a rib; however, the doctors assumed he was a victim of child abuse. There had been a program on TV the night before about battered children. They X-rayed Stephen and saw that he did not, in fact, have a broken bone. The cause of the crying was eventually diagnosed to be an earache. We were deliriously happy, not that he had an earache but there were no broken bones, and that the doctors were proven wrong in their suspicions.

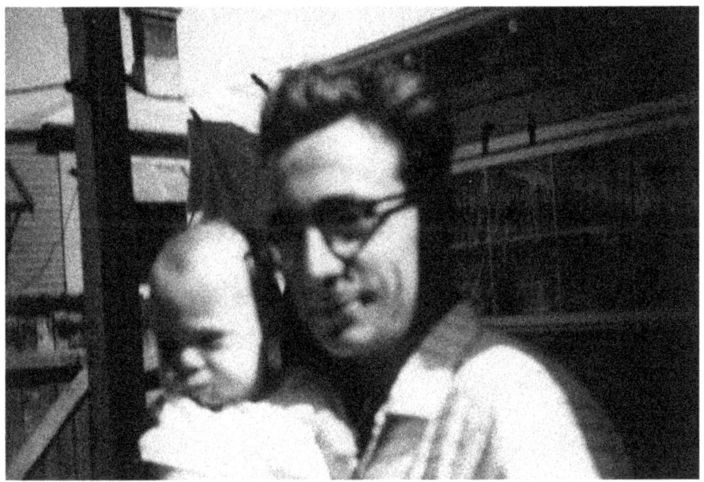

Stephen at 5 months with Ray, at the back of our house in South Fremantle

The perambulators (pram or baby carriage) of that time were made of heavy cane with a hood attached. When going anywhere on a bus, I had to lay my baby boy down on a blanket on the footpath, proceed to hook the pram onto the back of the bus, pick up my baby and then board the bus. On rare occasions, the bus driver would help. I now do not have the faintest idea how I managed to lift the heavy pram, given my own fragile bones, but I guess I had no other choice. Little did I realise I was in training for a lifetime of lifting wheelchairs and ramps as my child grew.

While bathing Stephen at seven months, he rolled off the kitchen table just as I reached down to pick up something from the floor.

Terrified, I gently lifted him up from the floor. To my amazement, he was not crying, and there were no broken bones. I felt overjoyed that he was smiling up at me. At that moment, I convinced myself again that Stephen was not going to be breaking his bones in the future. He was going to be okay. Denial was a wonderful address to reside at, bringing temporary respite from the callous truth – that Stephen would be at the mercy of this cruel disease all his life.

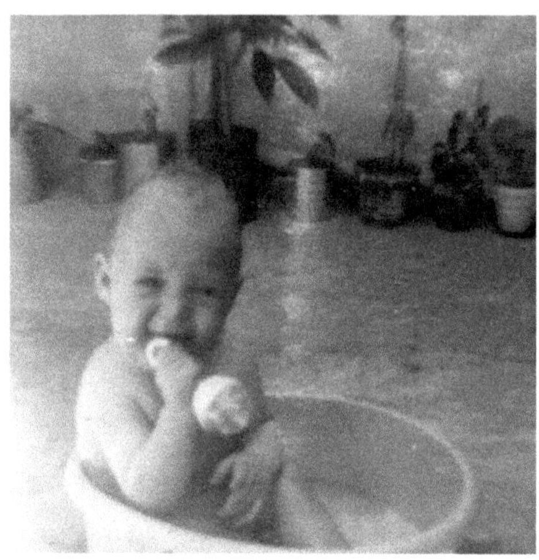

Stephen at 7 months

At this time, Ray was working as a cadet metallurgist in a steel foundry, as well as attending night school for a metallurgical degree. Ray knew he must be qualified to earn enough money to support and provide for a better future for his family.

Ray would come home from work around 4:00 PM to go to night school. Stephen and I would both be crying. Ray had to catch two buses to Perth in order to attend his courses. He would come back home around 10:00 PM, and Stephen and I would both still be crying. Ray would then take over nursing Stephen till they both fell asleep. Juggling work and a sick child with little sleep meant there was no time for Ray to study. The day of his final exam, he skimmed over his books. It was a mystery to me how he passed all final eight subjects and was awarded his Metallurgy Diploma.

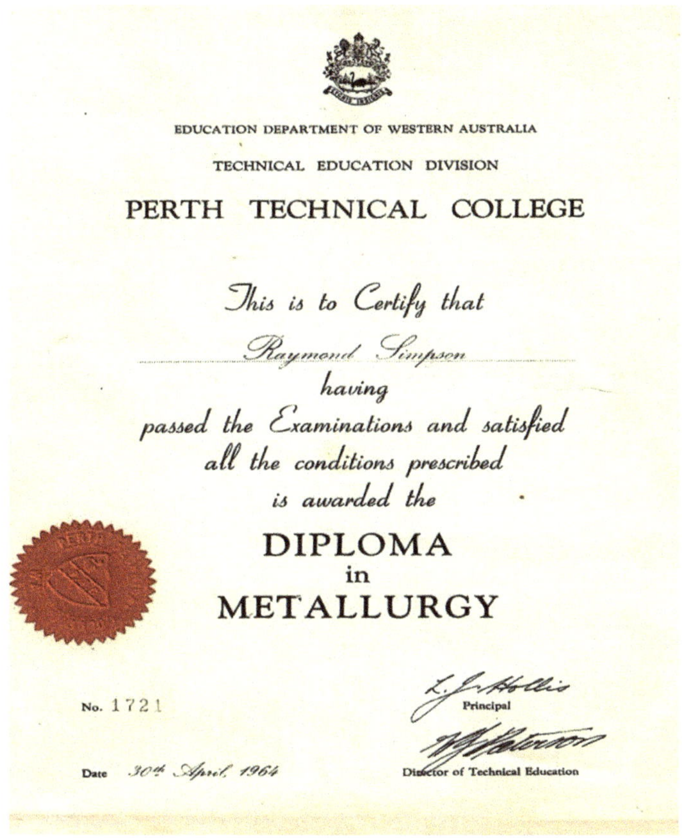
EDUCATION DEPARTMENT OF WESTERN AUSTRALIA

TECHNICAL EDUCATION DIVISION

PERTH TECHNICAL COLLEGE

This is to Certify that

Raymond Simpson

having

passed the Examinations and satisfied all the conditions prescribed

is awarded the

DIPLOMA
in
METALLURGY

No. 1721

Principal

Date *30th April 1964*

Director of Technical Education

Ray's Diploma in Metallurgy

Later, when we lived in the United States, Ray's diploma served to be invaluable and provided him with senior positions at many large organisations such as Utah Construction and Mining Company, Lucky Mac Uranium Mine in Wyoming, General Telephone and Electronics in Huntsville in Alabama, Homelite Chainsaws Manufacturing in Columbia in South Carolina, and General Electric and Hughes Tool Company in Houston in Texas.

3

Making Happy Memories

I often wonder now how we coped in the beginning. I think we were so young that we tenaciously clung to the hope that Stevie would be okay, and our situation would improve. We never turned to drugs or alcohol as many do when faced with extreme difficulties or painful situations; besides, there was no money left over for luxuries of any kind.

At this time, we had a black-and-white cat named Dinky. When Stephen was eight months old, he stood up in his cot hanging on to the rails, pointed down to Dinky on the floor and said his first word: "Dinkdoo!" Soon after, he started saying Mummy and Daddy and many other words. Of course, we were over the moon with pride that our little man was saying so many words as a baby. We proudly concluded it was a sign that our boy was going to be clever.

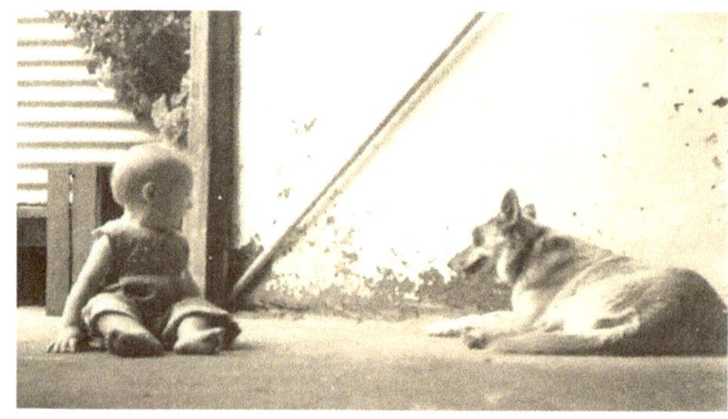

'A boy and his dog': Stephen aged 8½ months

At 10 months, Stephen developed the art form of perfectly feeding himself. He never missed his mouth or dropped any food from the spoon as small children are generally prone to do. However, on one occasion he was whimpering and turned the spoon around to a different angle to get the food in his mouth. In hindsight, we realised that his arm had been hurting due to a stress fracture.

Stephen took his first steps on my twenty-first birthday, May 22, 1961, when he was 13 months old. Ever since he was a toddler, Stephen's first love was playing with toy 'matchbox' cars. He would make dirt roads in the sand for them to run on. I loved to see him sitting for hours playing happily; it meant to me that he was safe as well.

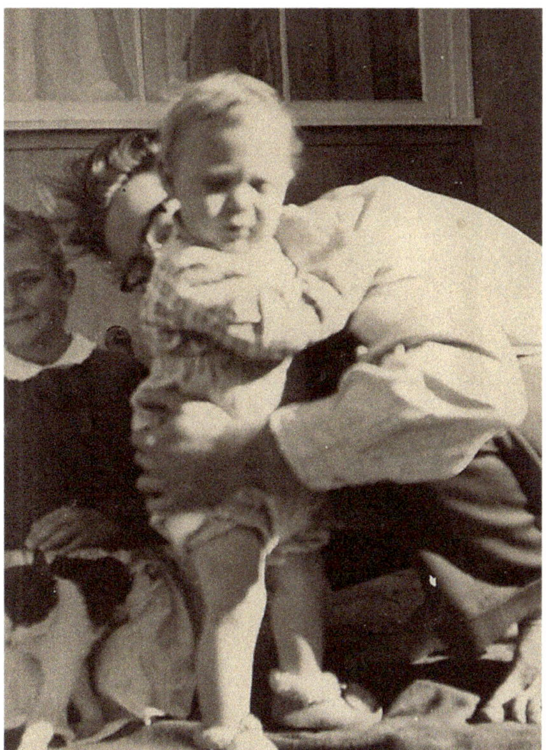

Stephen at 12 months with Ray and Dinky the cat, 1961

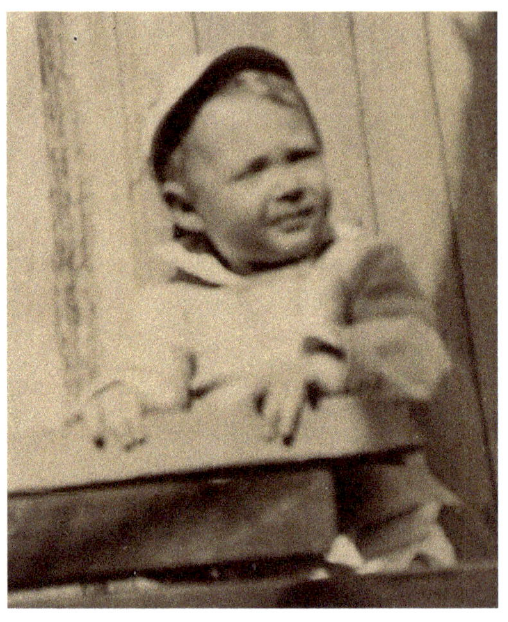

Stephen at 14 months, 1961

Later while he was learning to walk, he would often fall down and break an arm or a leg, requiring hospitalisations, X-rays and casts. This would become a never-ending cycle.

"Why? Why? Why?" I beseeched God. I prayed desperately to God, begging and pleading from the deepest part of my being for Him to heal my dear little boy, and then Stephen would break another bone soon after. I then came to the sad realisation that he would continue breaking his bones in the future. Since I had no signs or answers from God, I decided invariably that I was going to have to nurture and protect Stephen as best I could. I felt alone and frightened; I thought the more I could prevent fractures, the more I could protect him from unnecessary pain. I made up my mind to walk every step close behind him to catch him if he should stumble.

Knowing Stevie had so many challenges ahead, I kept hoping he would get better. I hovered over him constantly in order to protect him. I muddled through by never losing hope or faith that I, as his mother, could help him weather through his challenges.

Being young parents should have been a wondrous experience, watching a little baby grow and blossom and celebrating the developmental milestones. Every milestone Stephen reached, however, was overshadowed by which bone was currently broken and, in the future, morphed into which operation was scheduled next. I initially carefully documented every fracture to keep a comprehensive record. I stopped recording them when he was eight years old, as he had already suffered 300 fractures by that time. I was filling up the book and it was breaking my heart.

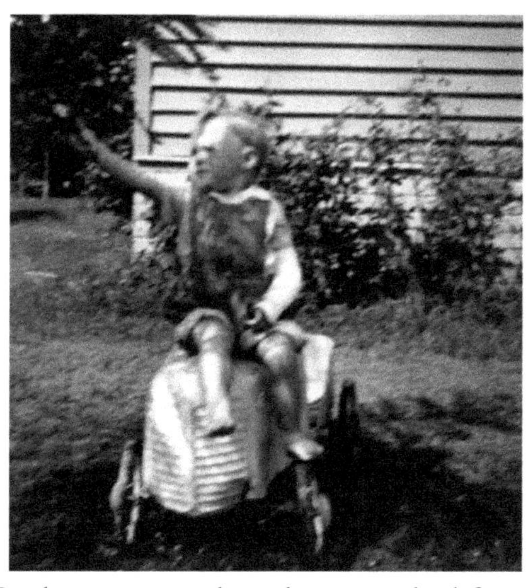

Stephen at 22 months with a cast on his left arm

Stephen's love for music was awakened soon after he started to walk. It came about one day by turning on the television to a show called Six O'Clock Rock featuring singer Johnny O'Keefe. The show started with the clock symbol showing Six O'Clock Rock – Time to Rock, and the music began with Johnny O'Keefe singing. Stephen would get up close to the television and begin dancing little steps to the music, having a great fun time. Stephen would also keenly listen to classical music that was always playing in our house. His love for all styles of music persisted throughout his life.

In 1962 we were living in South Fremantle, Western Australia. The little money we had was put away for Ray's night school fees, bus fares and baby food, and it was all we could afford as Ray had lost his job in the last year of his Diploma course. By chance, just before he was retrenched from his workplace, he bought a 100-kilogram bag of potatoes. That bag of potatoes was to feed us for the next nine months.

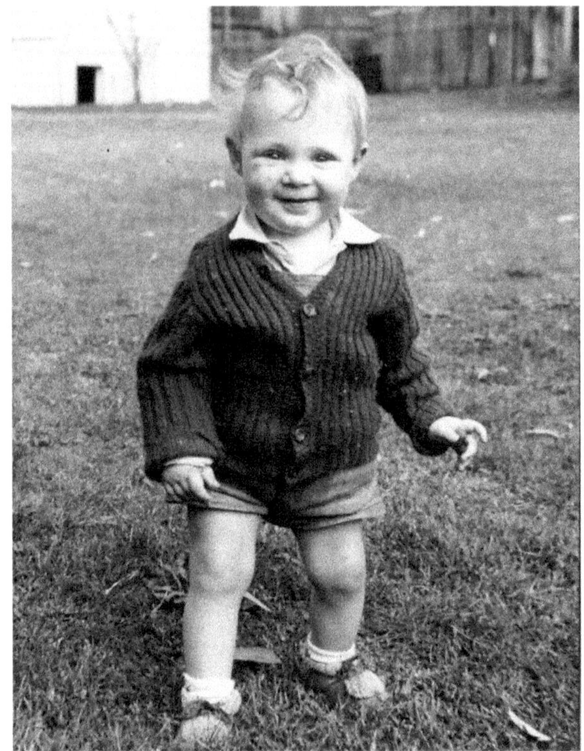

Stephen at 16 months with a cast on his right arm

I wonder how these days potatoes do not last more than a week without growing sprouts. Our menu back then consisted of a cycle of fried potatoes, boiled potatoes, baked potatoes, potato soup, scalloped potatoes, potato pie and mashed potatoes. I recall in a favourite movie Forrest Gump the many different ways for preparing 'Bubba Gump Shrimp'. We had just as many ways to cook potatoes. I became creative and served them night after night in a multitude of disguises. As a matter of necessity, I discovered how to make hamburger mince in many different guises as a form of gastronomic delight.

During these lean times, my mother and Ray's mother helped by bringing us bags of groceries, and she would slip some money to me as she left to cover any outstanding bills.

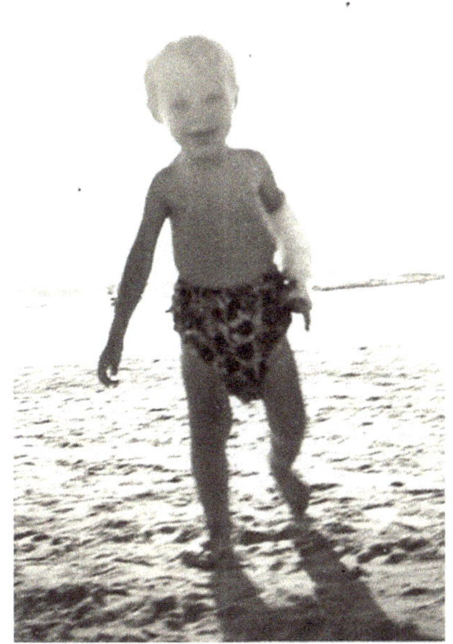

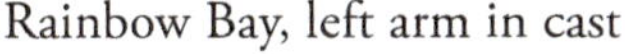

Rainbow Bay, left arm in cast

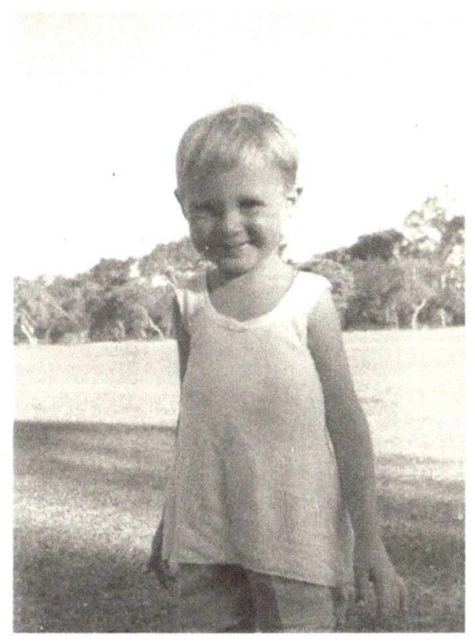

At the park, aged 3 years

When things looked grim, Ray and I would sit at the kitchen table wondering how we could solve our money problem. We would often decide to wait for the post in case some miracle arrived. On several occasions, my aunt in Queensland sent us $20, which would tide us over until the next emergency. I wondered if God was providing these miracles or if it was just a strange coincidence.

Stephen was extremely cute as a toddler, which made the bad times easy to forget. One day we came home from a visit to Ray's mother, and Stevie came in the back door and saw Dinky the cat sitting with eyes half-closed on the floor. Stevie crouched down on his little legs, put his arm gently around the cat's back, and while he and the cat looked at each other, said:

"Been on the choo-choo train, been on the bus, been to see Nana and now I'm home."

On another day at our house in South Fremantle, when Stephen was three years old, he went riding his tricycle on the footpath on our street. Ray walked in and asked, "Where's Stevie?"

"He went on the footpath on his trike," I replied.

Ray walked up the street looking for him. He came back and said he could not see Stevie anywhere. Just then, Stephen came to the back door.

"Where have you been?" Ray asked him. "I've been looking for you."

Stephen answered back cheerfully, "Did you find me, Dad?"

Picturing these and many other cherished memories helped sustain us through the battles ahead.

After that, we thought it a good idea to teach Stevie to memorise where he lived in case he ever got lost. We would ask him, "Where do you live?" and he would answer with, "160 Marine Terrace, South Freemumple [sic]." So cute.

We were proud of his ability to learn so quickly. He could also recite the day and month of his birth whenever we asked him.

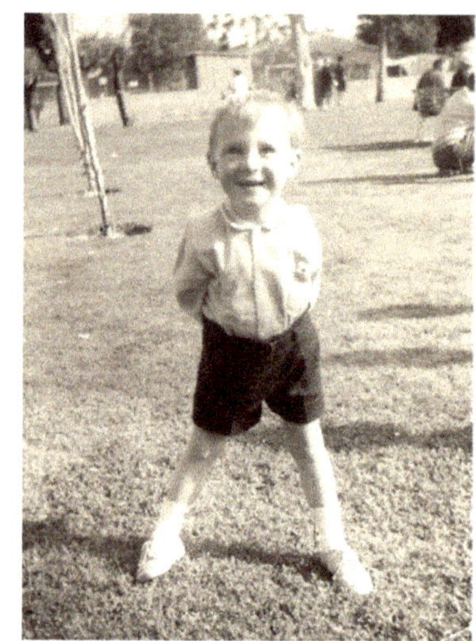

"Hello Daddy!": Stephen aged 3

In 1963, Ray was offered a metallurgical position at Whim Creek copper mine near Port Hedland, which was 1,650 km. north of Perth. We decided to move and start a new life there. We packed our belongings, borrowed $200 from Ray's aunt and caught a plane to Whim Creek. We were given a small house where we settled in comfortably.

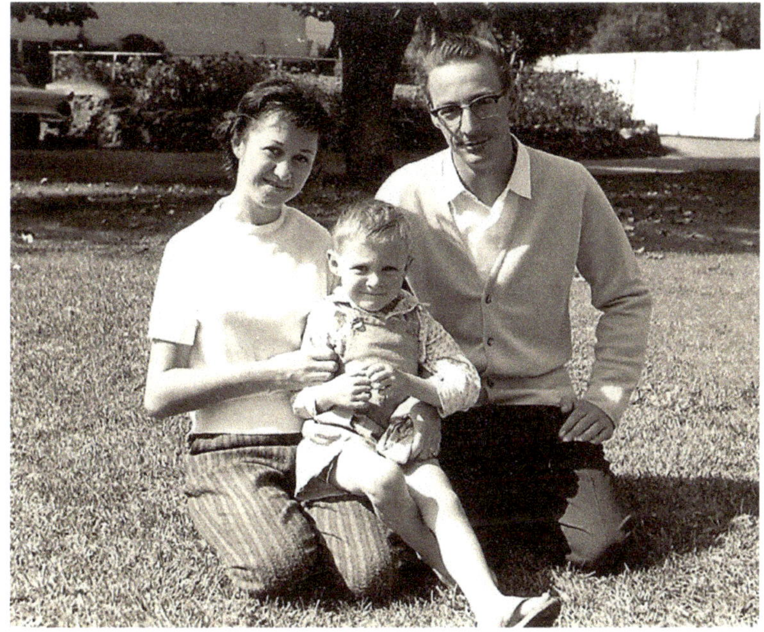

At the park: Stephen aged 3½, a rare photo with no casts

Not long after we moved, a truck driver stopped by the Whim Creek Hotel with a baby joey (kangaroo). He had come across a dead kangaroo on the road and found she had a joey about eighteen months old in her pouch. He stopped at the hotel with the joey and asked if anyone wanted it. Our family was happy together, but we always had room for additional members. It was not uncommon then for people living in rural areas to have pet kangaroos.

We brought the joey home and made her a bag pouch which we hung up on the wall. She was able to jump in and out of this pouch as if it was her mother's pouch. I fed her corn flour and milk to stop her getting scours or diarrhoea. We named her Popsey; I would call her by making clicking sounds like you do to communicate with horses, and she would come bouncing out and come to a dead stop at my feet. She followed us everywhere. She would sleep with us on our bed at night and finally became an integral family member. She enjoyed going fishing with us at Balla Balla near Whim Creek whenever it was possible for us to borrow a Land Rover and indulge in a recreational day.

The water in the tidal creek depended on the state of the tide and time. At low tide it was very shallow, and at other times it was very deep. We would wait till the creek was nearly filled and then park ourselves on the edge to fish for the treasures that had been brought in with the tide. This would often include large Western Australian salmon and delicious mud crabs.

The salmon we selected by size; those that we considered too large were returned to the water and those that protruded from a hessian bag were highly prized. It was not unusual to catch five or six premium-sized fish. We would donate the excess haul to other families in the small community.

Catching mud crabs was an entirely different scenario. This meant jiggling a long rod with a hook on the end down a hole in the creek bank. If a crab was hiding within the hole, the rod had to be twisted to get the hook behind the crab. The crab would be pulled out onto the bank and placed into the bag. Very few of these sweet-tasting delights were given away.

For Stephen, our fishing trips were a source of much fun and amusement. It was hilarious to watch Popsey hopping through the mud. On every third or fourth hop, the mud that had built up on her long legs and tail would throw her off balance. She would do a complete somersault, then stand up, shake herself and do it all over again. Sadly, our dear Popsey was mauled by a dog, an ending she did not deserve for all the joy and happiness she brought us.

During this time, the future started to look brighter. We felt less financial pressure as we finally had employment, money was

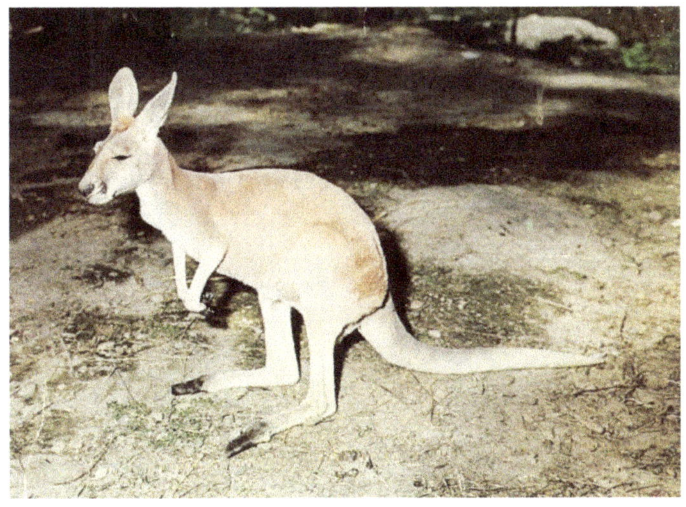

Popsey

coming in to pay bills and other things were on the menu rather than potatoes.

We were not there long when Stephen fell off his bed one day and broke his arm badly. Without thinking, I instinctively straightened his arm with my hands. Let me explain: when a bone breaks, it takes a few seconds for the sharp pain of the break to be felt, and putting the bone back in a natural position alleviates the acute pain just a little. I was always quick to react to Stephen's distress.

We headed off to Port Hedland Hospital, a drive of about 100 miles or 160 kilometres, with me holding his painful arm all the way. In those days, the roads were not sealed and the corrugations made a bumpy ride, adding to Stephen's pain.

As we were waiting in the hospital, a very obese woman came to the desk and Stephen, even though his broken arm was very painful, tugged gently on my sleeve and whispered, "Mum, why is that lady in a big dress?" Stephen saw a big dress and not a big lady, a testament to the wonderful way a child's mind works.

At the hospital I was always calm; however, once we were home, I would always shake uncontrollably after such episodes.

In the small community where we lived, there were only three or four women I could socialise with. I loved helping out in the hotel kitchen with the wife of the proprietor. She had the help of a lovely Aboriginal woman named Lena, who called me 'Missy'. One morning I was trying to light the old stove with newspaper and some small pieces of firewood. I threw in some kerosene and bent down to blow onto the twigs, and all of a sudden it ignited and blew out onto my face, singing my hair and eyebrows. Lena screamed, "Missy, Missy!" and quickly wrapped a towel around my head. I looked quite a sight without my eyebrows and part of my hair burnt and moulded into lumps.

Summer temperatures there were frequently above 40°C (105°F), and nearby Marble Bar held the record of 160 consecutive days above these temperatures. The land was harsh, but people of the outback were tougher. Many are the stories told of the old-time prospectors wheeling their worldly possessions in a wheelbarrow through this harsh country in search of the elusive gold.

Washing dishes as fast as I could after the evening meal would leave a pool of water from my body sweating profusely in the heat. The nights brought little relief. One night I had just dozed off to sleep when I thought there was a spider running across my back. I leaped out of bed screaming. We stripped the bed looking for the spider but there was none to be seen. Still, it happened again as soon as I nodded off to sleep. I decided to be brave and wallop it hard when I felt it running across my back. To my amazement, I felt only my back drenched in perspiration.

The mine was going well. It had been operated by Germans early in the century and at the outbreak of the First World War, the Germans had been interned and the mine closed down. Then in 1963, the Japanese re-opened the mine in defiance of the Immigration Law. When the mine was operating smoothly, an enterprising opportunist took the company to court under provision of Australia's White Australia policy. This effectively precluded persons of non-Anglo-Saxon heritage from residing in Australia and resulted in each individual Japanese person being fined the equivalent of $10 and each being granted permission to stay in Australia for two years.

This change in the Immigration Law ultimately led to the exploration and development of the massive iron ore deposits in the adjacent desert areas, the delivery railway lines, and the huge harbours necessary to accommodate the 250,000 tonne vessels needed to carry the precious cargo to Japan. However, it also resulted in the almost immediate closure of the mine, which meant Ray was again unemployed.

We flew back to Perth for new opportunities but found that jobs were scarce, and we missed the sunshine and high wages of working above the 26th parallel (the tropic of Capricorn) which had tremendous tax breaks due to the harsh weather conditions. We longed to go back.

4

Moving Up North

Our only chance to resume this rugged lifestyle was to buy a used car and head north into the unknown and search for work in the small mines that dotted the area.

We borrowed $50 from an aunt and returned to Whim Creek, leaving Stephen temporarily in the care of Ray's mother.

At the Whim Creek Hotel, we were offered food and lodgings in return for being short-term publicans while the owners went on holiday.

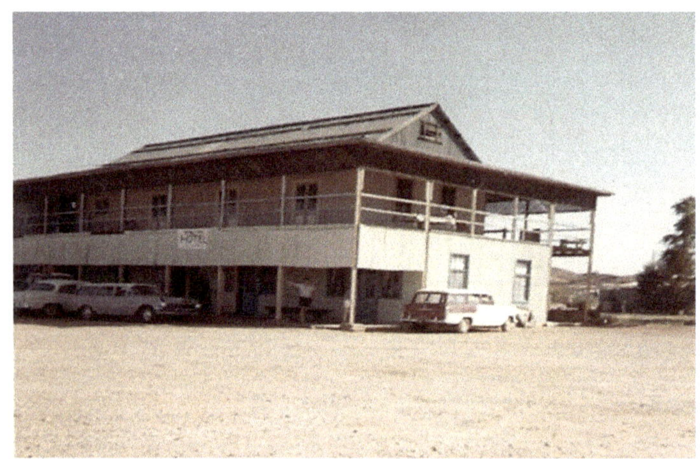

Whim Creek Hotel and our first car, a red-and-white station wagon

For the next six weeks, we ran that hotel like clockwork. Because of its remote location, it was mostly quiet with an intermittent flurry of activity when customers arrived, mainly truck drivers carrying perishables to markets in the North West. Ray served the beers while I served copious canned curried-sausage sandwiches and canned steak-and-onion sandwiches made with fried bread. The patrons loved these simple delicacies. Word quickly spread between the truckies and business boomed.

An opportunity came up at Port Hedland where Ray and I both obtained employment – Ray in an engineering capacity and I with secretarial duties at Utah Construction and Mining Company, an American firm that was building the Mt Goldsworthy Iron Ore Mine in Port Hedland.

We gladly welcomed our new employment positions. Now that we had stability of income and accommodation, we were able to have Stephen return to the family fold. He flew as an unaccompanied child on the DC3, which then serviced the small towns in the Northwest of the state. We rented a house, and our car provided mobility in a town where public transport was non-existent.

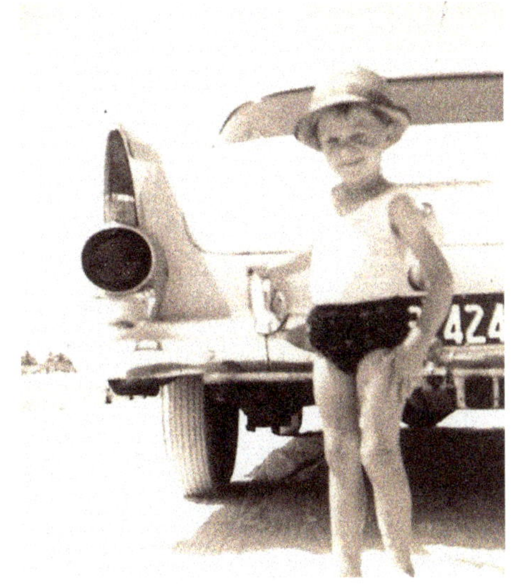

A sunny day in Port Hedland: Stephen aged 3½

During Christmas 1964, Utah Construction and Mining Company threw a wonderful and generous Christmas party for its employees and their families, with presents from Santa for all the children. One of our American friends, who took a photo of Stephen receiving his gift from Santa, said to us, "You have got to see this (photo), Stevie looks like a little diplomat!"

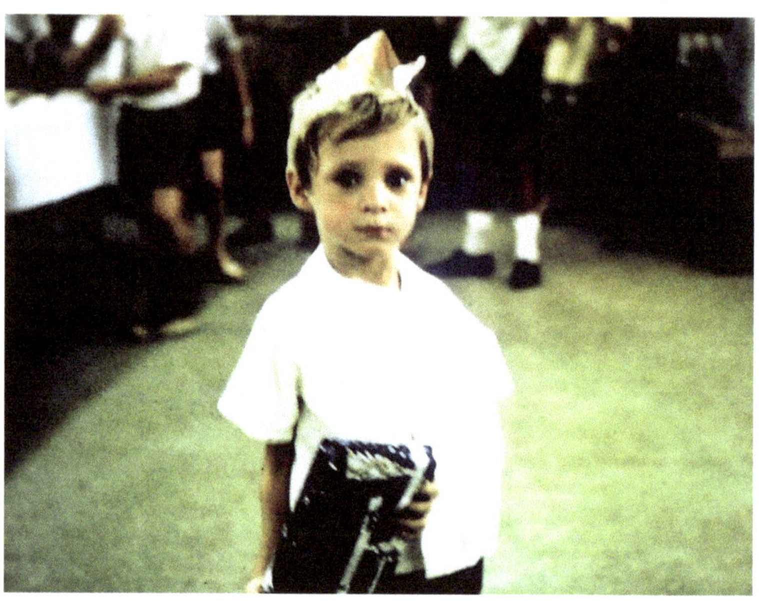

Stevie with his present from Santa and sling on left arm, Christmas 1964

We were now showing progress from previous hard times. Stephen was still able to walk and attended first grade at Port Hedland Primary School. Every day I asked him what he had learnt, and he often answered that he played with rods. I was concerned that Stephen was not learning anything and was just playing with rods every day. I paid a visit to his school and found out it was not the usual kind of game – Cuisenaire rods are learning aids that provide a hands-on way to explore and learn mathematical concepts. I was quickly reassured that Stephen was getting the right tuition in mathematics, a subject for which he quickly developed a lifelong love.

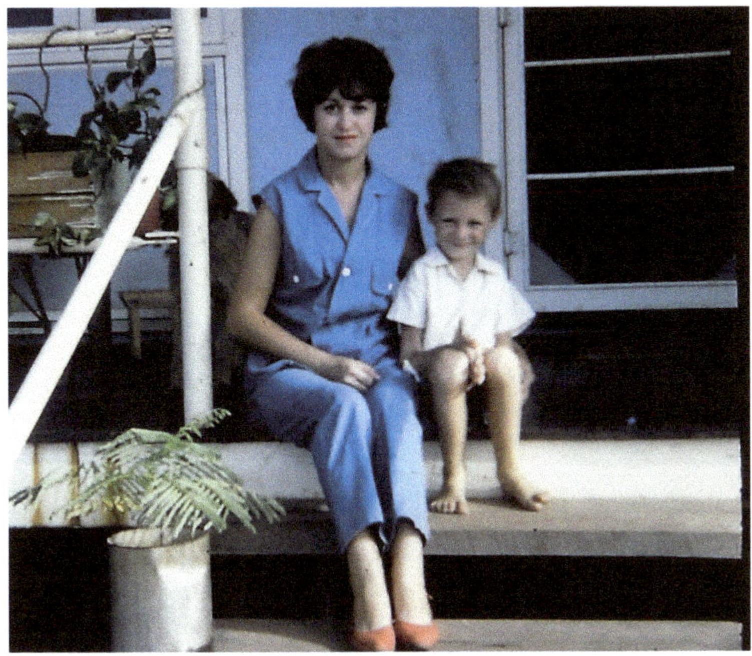

Me and Stephen in Port Hedland, 1965

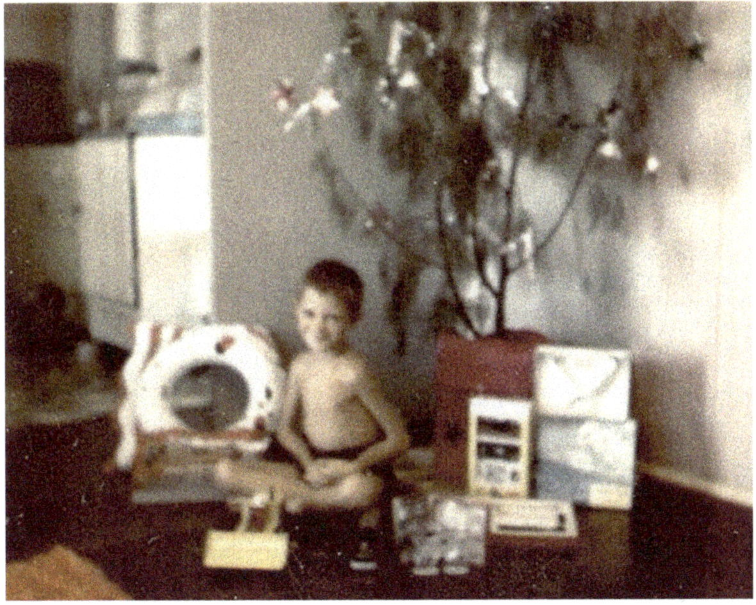

Christmas with Stephen under the she-oak tree, 1965

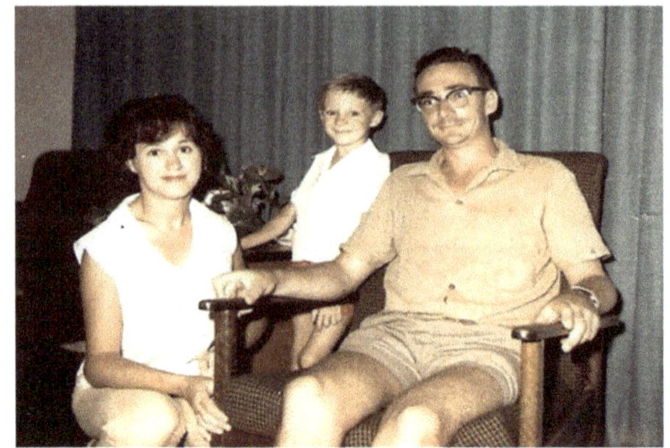

In our house in Port Hedland, 1965

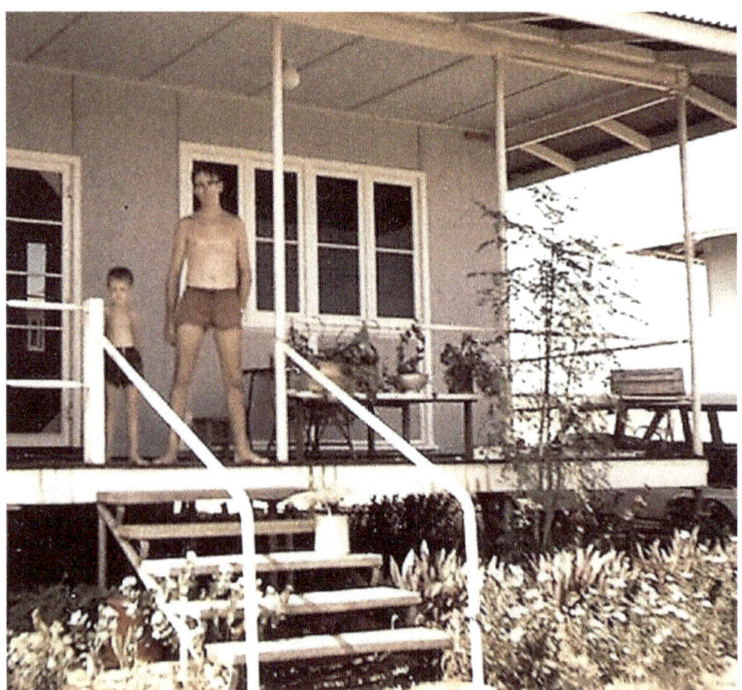

Ray and Stephen in Port Hedland, 1965

Through Ray's work we met the Hendricks, an American family with two little girls, Robin and Vicki. We had lots of fun with them on fishing excursions and often took turns cooking Australian and American meals. Their two little girls and Stephen played by emulating family life within our household. They would mimic Ray and I by playing mummies-and-daddies with Stephen on the front porch. Robin, the elder girl, would be the mum, and Vicki the dad. Stephen would be the baby. They would wrap Stephen up in bandages.

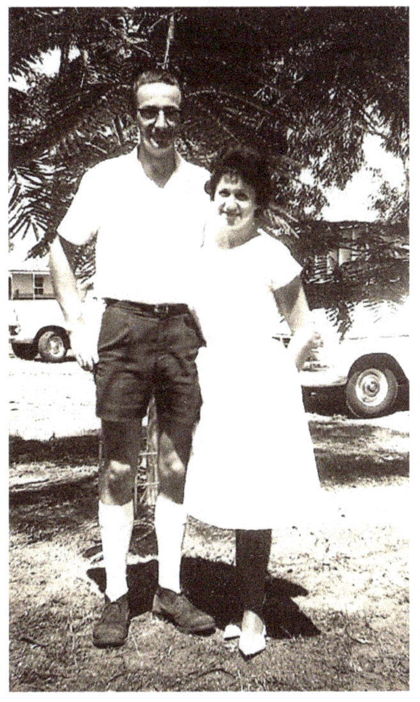

Ray and me working in Port Hedland, 1966

On school days I would pick up Robin and the three of us would sing songs merrily all the way to their school: *The Big Ship Sails on the Alley Alley Oh* and *Oh Be Careful Little Eyes What You See.*

In January 1967, Port Hedland was hit by a tropical storm. Within 24 hours, it produced 15 inches (381 mm) of rain. I had to pick Ray up from the mine camp site. I carried Stephen into the car, with our dog Butch following close at my heels, and drove through rain like a waterfall, without any idea what was going to happen next. Through blinding rain, we reached the mine camp site and Ray ran out towards us and quickly jumped into the car. While driving slowly back on the saturated muddy road, an adjacent 20,000-gallon water storage tank built on a 40-foot (12-metre) tower collapsed without any prior warning; the ground beneath it had been undermined by the deluge of water pouring off the elevated platform.

We looked up and saw a huge mountain of water and sand rapidly cascading towards us. We all thought we were going to be washed down the cliff and die. I was resigned to my fate and felt no fear, and I wondered later if that is how you feel when you are about to die. When the wave of sand and water hit us, the car stopped dead, engulfed in sand up to the windscreen. Then out of the black night, we saw car headlights coming up the hill towards us. Since our car doors were blocked by sand and could not be opened, we had to climb out the windows. Handing Stevie carefully out through the window while ignoring the downpour was a unique and tense operation.

We made our way with Ray carrying Stephen with one arm and pulling me towards the headlights with the other. Fortunately, it was a taxi driver on his way to pick up someone from the camp site; however, he could not get through due to the sand and water making the road impassable. We implored him to take us as passengers instead, and while he agreed, he did not wish for our wet dog to get into his taxi. Standing in the drenching rain, Ray pleaded with him to have mercy on the dog, noting that we were stranded in a remote part of Western Australia, and it was raining torrents late at night. Eventually, the taxi driver grudgingly agreed to take the dog. Much to his horror, as soon as Butch jumped into the car, he shook his wet coat vigorously, and mud and water was flung in every direction in his pristine taxi.

When we arrived home, we reluctantly paid an extra $5 to clean the taxi.

The next day it took five hours to extricate our car using heavy mining machinery. Further work was required to get the car started, and we headed for the nearest service station to have the erratic steering checked. The service man drove the car out of sight and hosed down the wheel caps to remove sand, which was making the wheels unbalanced. He charged us $40 – almost half a week's wages – for five minutes' work.

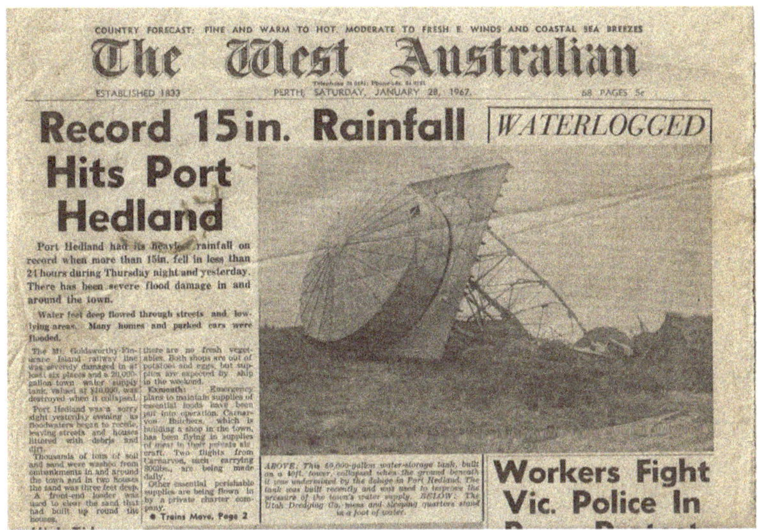

COUNTRY FORECAST: FINE AND WARM TO HOT. MODERATE TO FRESH E. WINDS AND COASTAL SEA BREEZES

The West Australian

ESTABLISHED 1833 | PERTH, SATURDAY, JANUARY 28, 1967. | 68 PAGES 5c

Record 15in. Rainfall Hits Port Hedland

Port Hedland had its heaviest rainfall on record when more than 15in. fell in less than 24 hours during Thursday night and yesterday. There has been severe flood damage in and around the town.

Water feet deep flowed through streets and low-lying areas. Many homes and parked cars were flooded.

The Mt. Goldsworthy-Finucane Island railway line was severely damaged in at least six places and a 20,000-gallon town water supply tank, valued at $10,000, was destroyed when it collapsed.

Port Hedland was a sorry sight yesterday evening as floodwaters began to recede, leaving streets and houses littered with debris and dirt.

Thousands of tons of soil and sand were washed from embankments in and around the town and in two houses the sand was three feet deep.

A front-end loader was used to clear the sand that had built up round the houses.

... there are no fresh vegetables. Both shops are out of potatoes and eggs, but supplies are expected by ship in the weekend.

Exmouth: Emergency plans to maintain supplies of essential foods have been put into operation. Carnarvon Butchers, which is building a shop in the town, has been flying in supplies of meat in their private aircraft. Two flights from Carnarvon, each carrying 800lbs., are being made daily.

Other essential perishable supplies are being flown in by a private charter company.

• Trains Move, Page 2

WATERLOGGED

ABOVE: This 60,000-gallon water-storage tank, built on a 40ft. tower, collapsed when the ground beneath it was undermined by the deluge in Port Hedland. The tank was built recently and was used to improve the pressure of the town's water supply. BELOW: The Utah Dredging Co. mess and sleeping quarters stand in a foot of water.

Workers Fight Vic. Police In

Newspaper clipping about extreme rainfall in Port Hedland, January 1967

The climate in general was hot and humid, but the evenings were usually pleasant. Air conditioning did not exist except in the offices of the American companies. Wide casement windows with attached flyscreens and ceiling fans were the only concessions to the tropical climate.,

The beer gardens of the two hotels in Port Hedland, The Pier and The Esplanade were always popular, particularly on Saturday nights, as Sunday was the only day off in the 60-hour a week regime. This was the early days of the satellites and they were clearly visible to the patrons of the outdoor beer gardens. The American satellites travelled from east to west, and the Russian ones from north to south; it was not uncommon to count a total of 26 tracks across the evening sky even without the advantage of having had a few drinks!

The town was covered in a veneer of reddish-purple dust from the earth-moving operations associated with the construction of the railroad and harbour needed for the export of the iron ore. The ore contained 63% iron and was eagerly sought by steel smelters as direct blast furnace feed. Consequently, laundry day was selected in accordance with the direction of the hot, dry wind. Many a clothesline full of laundry was rendered a dark pink hue when the wind changed direction.

I came home from work one day to see a 'black' man chopping wood in the yard. I initially thought it was some nice man doing me a favour, but as I got nearer, I saw it was my husband Ray, who probably had just come from work. He was so completely covered in the reddish-purple dust that I had mistaken him for a kind Aboriginal man chopping my wood. We laughed as Ray looked at himself and conceded that my mistake was entirely plausible.

Stephen, meanwhile, was progressing well at school. He enjoyed playing with Robin and Vicki Hendricks, who by then had been joined by a new baby sister named Dove. Their parents were extremely proud and referred to the new baby as their little Aussie. We would often socialise with the Hendricks family and were frequent dinner guests at their very modern, comfortably air-conditioned and employer-provided three-bedroom house. It was there we learned to eat our steak medium-rare as opposed to overcooked, dry and tough. When the project finished and they had to return to America, we were sad to see them leave, little knowing that our paths would cross again in the not-too-distant future.

One day Stephen came home from school and asked me for five cents. When I asked him why, he said he wanted to buy a light bulb from his friend a few doors from our house. I gave him five cents and he came back with a light bulb whose wire element was broken. Stephen was happy and convinced he had purchased a bargain. We were amused by this but cautioned him to check any future 'bargains' thoroughly before paying for them.

When the school holidays arrived, Stephen, then aged six years, flew from Port Hedland to Perth under the guiding eye of a hostess to stay with Ray's mother.

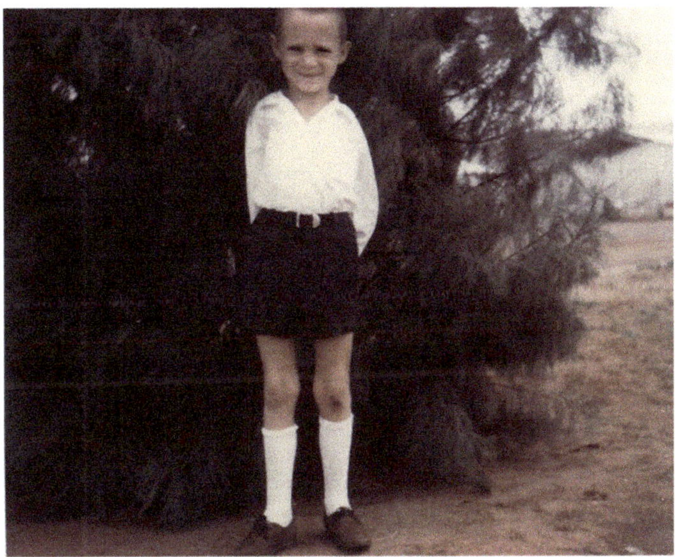

Stephen going on holiday from Port Hedland to Perth, aged 6

His Nana later recalled how she once told him to sit up on bed for being a naughty boy for swearing. Stephen had sat on his bed rocking back and forth with his stuffed toys Teddy and Mickey Mouse, singing his own composition to the tune of Here we go round the Mulberry Bush:

"How can I kill me bloody old Nana; how can I kill me bloody old Nana."

His Nana came to the door and was watching him sing when Stephen, noticing her out of the corner of his eye, broke into the correct words quickly without missing a beat:

"Here we go round the mulberry bush; here we go round the mulberry bush."

Ray's mother had to step back where he could not see her laughing; she laughed so much that tears ran down her face.

Around this time, Stephen broke his left arm. The doctor wanted to put a rod in his radius – the long bone joining the elbow and wrist – because he thought it would keep Stephen's arm from continually breaking. The operation, sadly, was not a success due to the bone being flat and ribbon-shaped and having virtually no channel to put in the rod. During the operation, the doctor had to hunt around and find a piece of wire to put into the bone as the rod was too thick. Stephen's left arm was never the same again. It was further weakened due to the trauma of surgery. His arm did not grow after that and had to be supported with a brace for years. It was one of his worst surgical outcomes.

Many similar scenarios followed in the years to come, of limbs being operated on with poorer-than-before results. Out of the 47 operations Stephen underwent, three-quarters had negative outcomes. With every surgery we hoped in vain that this one would be successful, but that seldom happened. His overall condition was not improving.

The Americans Ray worked with at Utah Construction suggested we immigrate to the USA, based on Ray's Diploma in Metallurgy. We were excited by the possibility of getting better treatment for Stephen in America. The process entailed a year of paperwork with the American Embassy to obtain the necessary sponsorship and documentation to work in the USA. Meanwhile, the construction phase of the Mt Goldsworthy mine was nearing practical completion, and Ray was selected to commission the huge crushing and screening plant at the mine site. At the completion of commissioning, Ray was due to be transferred, at our cost, to a uranium mine in Riverton, Wyoming.

During our time in Port Hedland, Ray was a regular contributor to a mimeographed weekly newsletter under the pseudonym Laury Ett.

He wrote verses poking fun at various aspects of life in a country town, plagued by flies, dogs and dust. On learning of his imminent transfer to Wyoming USA, Ray penned a final submission, at last revealing the identity of the scribe who had provided cynical amusement to the local residents.

19.4.67.

THE VIEWS OF A MUSE

"It seems to me, I've heard folk say,
The local winds blow the wrong way,
And shower us with clouds of dust,
-A crude, barbaric form of rust.
Perhaps that company could sink,
Their iron ore in molten zinc,
And then before they'd realized,
The iron would be galvanized.
Or then again, to beat the nags,
Seal it up in plastic bags,
As the Government, tongue in cheek,
Forced the owners of Whim Creek.
"No dust allowed" the water sprays,
Sprayed on and on for many days,
No rock could fall from off the belt,
Big Brother made his presence felt.
When we changed an act of Parliament
(which was the reason they were sent)
The owners quietly slipped away,
To come again another day.
In them, alas! we'd put our trust,
And now they shower us with dust,
But don't despair, all is not lost,
Our Government will not be bossed.
We'll see them act! They'll not be meek!
(They'll hide and turn the other cheek!)
Or then again, they may relent,
And cut in half our lofty rent.
To compensate the cost of power,
Which we burn for hour on hour,
To keep our houses clean and neat,
To pur the dust back on the street.
Where easterlies from down the track
Will pick it up and blow it back,
Onto the Isle of Finucane,
And then we'll get it back again!
And so good souls, please grin and bear it,
You may as well, you darn well wear it,
Remember this, and I'll be terse,
It's going to be a damn sight worse!
The Newman crowd will soon anoint
With iron ore our Nelson Point,
There is perhaps just one outlet,
We must put pressure on the Met.
For to escape this ghastly pall,
They must not send a wind at all.
These then, Sir, are just my views,
Perhaps they'll suit the "Hedland News".

LAURY ETT.

EDITOR:
Laury Ett's views don't necessarily suit the "Hedland News" but as the Poem displays great imagination and iron (ical) humour, I could hardly not print it. I only hope that the "powers that be" will accept it with equal good will. In relation to this dust problem, the following quotations were passed to me during the last week:

26/4/1967

TERSE VERSES.

In Moore Street in the light of day,
You can hear a Mantis pray,
In Moore Street of a midnight, dark,
Forty million mongrels bark

****

The Manganese goes to and fro
No matter where the breezes blow,
It must be costly; half each load,
Ends up lying on the road.

****

I hope among the Newman starters,
There comes a firm like Charlie Carters,
To Lower prices day by day,
That I might bank some of my pay.

****

I never thought I'd live to see
An iron coated, purple tree ,
Indeed unless we lay this pall,
We soon won't see a tree at all.

****

Laury Ett.

(How about a few verses on
'The Road to Pretty Pool' Laury : Editor)

ODE TO PRETTY POOL

When I was young, I like a fool
Took the road to Pretty Pool
And having lately seen the track
I think I'd better put it back.
I drove out there the other day
A tourist with me, by the way,
We bounced around and slid and tossed,
I thought my sump and diff. I'd lost
But the part we liked the best,
The bulldust holes above the crest.
We scattered dust both far and wide,
And scrambled out the other side.
We went into the rooms to change,
And smelt an odour somewhat strange,
In booming region of great wealth,
Such monuments to Public Health!
The local council's revenue,
Has much increased last year or two,
So much so, despite my greetings,
They hide the Minutes of the meetings.
Their money from our motor cars,
And speeders (in our public bars?)

Should be spent with zest and zeal
On giving us a better deal,
And seal the road to our resort,
Where we all go to have our sport,
Or loll about on golden sands,
(First removing all the cans),
And open up our own stocks, cool,
Beside our local swimming pool,
And making comments, seldom witty,
About the man who named it "PRETTY".

LAURY ETT.

"THE SAGA OF LAURY ETT"

Act iv.
"I'm sorry, but I've been away
On a visit to King Bay,
There to scream and rave and rant,
To supervise the Pellet Plant.
And thanks to these pep talks of mine,
That project will be done on time,
But now I'm safely back again,
And taking up my poison pen,
I'll compose some verse for you,
Cause I have little else to do.

---oOo---

Act v.
Now I've been told with great elan,
I cannot see the Council's plan,
This tickles me, for, what a blow !
I saw it several weeks ago.
And that's the truth, for what it's worth,
I saw the crazy thing in Perth.
No more will sultry sirens vamp
From portals at the two mile camp,
They're shifting it (Oh! taxis; drool)
Out by the road to Pretty Pool,
This move is wise, I must explain,
For who'd be happy when a train,
All loaded up with Iron Ore,
Comes screaming through their kitchen door?

---oOo---

Act vi.
Another thing that made me frown,
The placing of our brand new town!
No water here, or roads or light,
To guide my footsteps home at night!
Now here's a thing I'd like to do!
To show the "brains" a thing or two,
I'd write a note and thus infer
They have a look at Dampier!
This modern town, so trim, so neat,
With homes of brick on ev'ry street,
And rent so low it is a farce
Airconditioned; tinted glass
Fully furnished, plus garage
The brains would say "It's a mirage".
And specify those paradoxes;
Asbestos castles called hot boxes,
Their choice of sites, I feel is strange,
Right within the Airport's range.
The screaming turbines late at night
Would even put a ghost to flight,
And first off in the brand new city
There'll be an Anti-Noise Committee,

. 3 .. 17.5.67.

With deputations thick and fast,
Who'll be ignored as in the past,
But battle on; do not relent
You may get into Parliament
Where in time your turn will come
To turn deaf ears to everyone,
And when in doubt or low on luck
Join the game of "Pass the Buck,
And to your leaders' speech enthrall
Never thinking for yourselves at all."

---oOo---

FINALE

"And now's the time with much regret,
We announce the end of Laury Ett,
I hope we all have had some fun,
Without upsetting anyone,
For now I'm off to cram my cranium,
With exciting facts about Uranium.
I'm shortly off to U.S.A.
So that is all from Simpson: Ray.

RAYMOND SIMPSON

EDITOR:

Thanks a lot, Ray, for your excellent contributions. I think you may have upset some "just a little", but in general your criticisms have been appreciated and much looked-forward to.
Best of luck in the future,
From "MOST OF PORT HEDLAND."

PART 2: LEARNING THE AMERICAN WAY

STEPHEN AGE 7—14

5

Going to America

In July 1967, with three suitcases, we set out on a new adventure to Riverton, Wyoming. We were excited at the prospect of seeing America and optimistic for new treatments for our boy. Physically, we moved over 10,000 miles or 16,000 km away, but to our surprise, we made a bigger move culturally. Going from one English-speaking country to another, one may think that the differences would be subtle, but we encountered a lot more than we had expected. In those days, there was not the same influx of news into Australia about America, and prior to our departure we knew very little except for the fact that we were going to a land of new opportunities.

On our way to Wyoming, we chose to stop in Hawaii and San Francisco. We arrived in Hawaii on July 7, 1967. There were still celebrations going on for the Fourth of July, the American Independence Day. This was our first cultural adjustment with the American accent all around us. We were amazed that the police wore guns, batons and handcuffs. Australian police at that time were unarmed.

The first meal we had in Hawaii was a hot dog, covered in ketchup, onions and pinto beans on a soft bread bun. It was the most delicious hot dog one could imagine. Usually, Stephen did not have a big appetite and ate painfully slowly, but even he gobbled up that hot dog with haste.

The next wondrous adventure for us was ordering a meal at a restaurant. We studied the menu and ordered 'roast lamb dinner' since it sounded the simplest. To our amazement, the waitress asked us what dressing we would like to have on the salad. "We don't have salad with a roast," we said dubiously, and the waitress replied, "A salad comes with every meal." So, we obediently ate the salad as an entrée before the roast. We quickly adjusted to the American cuisine, and to this day we still always have a salad with our evening meal.

We flew to San Francisco on the 10th July for the familiarisation interview with Utah Construction and Mining Company personnel. Ray had to get induction paperwork for employment with Lucky Mac Uranium Mine located 53 miles (85 km) from Riverton, Wyoming. One of the men from the company drove us over the Golden Gate Bridge, resplendent in bright, sunny weather. On the return trip fifteen minutes later, however, a dense fog had rolled in and totally obscured all but the lower level of the bridge. This is almost a daily occurrence, we later realised; therefore, morning viewing is generally best. Seeing for the first time the magnificent bridges and numerous overpasses in America was mind-boggling to us, and an endless source of fascination for Stephen. Later, when we developed our photos, most showed only overpasses and bridges.

As we returned to our hotel in San Francisco, we were surprised at the number of signs indicating fall-out shelters. The populace had been bombarded with 'cold war' messages about the probability of a nuclear attack, and numerous buildings were designated as refuges. We later learned that backyard nuclear shelters could be readily purchased, although no guarantee was available with regard to their effectiveness. The threat of nuclear attack was prominent in the lives of the American public for many years.

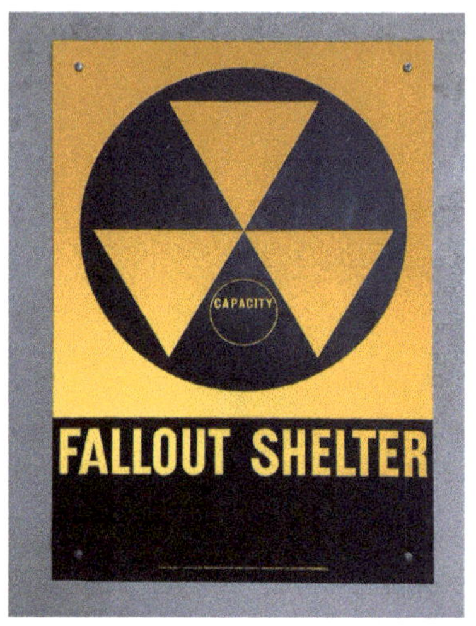

Fallout Shelter signs were everywhere in USA, 1967

We finally boarded our flight on the 12th July to take us to our new home in Riverton, Wyoming. We flew over the Rocky Mountains, which were still covered in snow, and marvelled at the view through our airplane window. When we landed, it seemed the snow-capped peaks were all around us. We were met by the Mine Manager and whisked off to a motel, which was to be our home until we found a rental residence.

America was so vastly different from rural Australia, especially the small-town population of Port Hedland where we came from. We were amazed by everything. The size of the cars was enormous; we saw huge Cadillacs, Chevrolets, Mercury's and Buicks parked in the streets. They seemed so long from the front to the back and had huge fins and grilles. Stephen's favourites were the Corvette Stingray and the Mustang.

We rented our first house in Riverton, Wyoming, at 802 E Jackson on the Wind River Shoshone Reservation. Only a day after we settled in, a neighbour knocked on our door with a cake to welcome us to the neighbourhood. One by one the neighbours came by to meet us and welcome us to America. The Welcome Wagon movement was highly active in Wyoming, with total strangers appearing with hot meals and maps of the area, where shopping centres, schools and churches were all clearly identified. They even told us about community Bingo games. In the first game we went to, Stephen won $90. This was a significant sum of money in those days, equivalent to about a week of Ray's salary. At the time we were low on finances, waiting for Ray's first pay cheque. We used Stephen's winnings for various necessities and promised to pay him back.

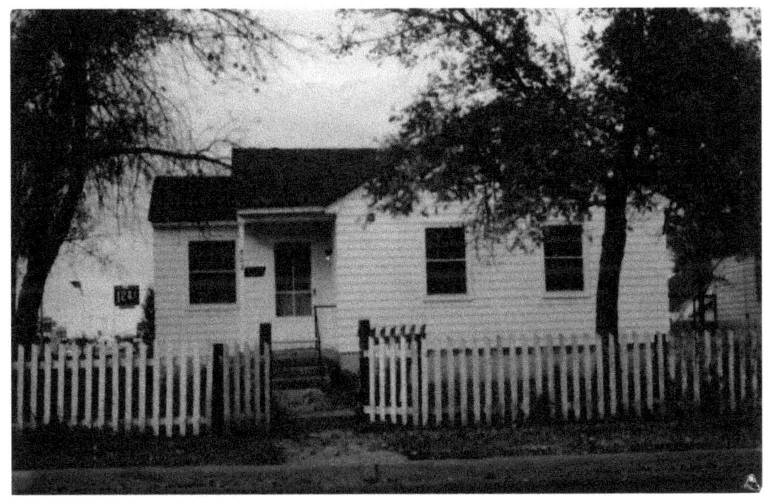

Our first house, 802 East Jackson, Riverton, Wyoming

Within two weeks of Ray commencing employment at the mine, several Shriner members contacted the Shriners organisation in Salt Lake City, Utah, to see if Stephen would be eligible for free treatment at their hospitals. The Shriners were graduates of the Freemason fraternity who, in 1922, decided to actively assist crippled children and opened the first orthopaedic hospital in Shreveport, Louisiana. By 1967, there were many hospitals across the USA providing free treatment for children suffering burns, cleft palates, spinal injuries and other orthopaedic conditions.

Two weeks later, we found ourselves on a plane to Salt Lake City, heading for an assessment at the hospital. The airfare, accommodation and taxis were all paid for by the local Shriners. After visiting the hospital, Ray went into an auto dealership and tried to negotiate for a vehicle. Our prospects were very grim, particularly when the dealership manager asked about Ray's credit record. He didn't have one, but he had his pay cheque details in his wallet and the manager accepted this as proof of gainful employment and allowed us to purchase a vehicle.

The next day, we drove back to Riverton and introduced the local population to the first TOYOTA to be seen in the area. We had had experience with these cars in the outback and knew they were both reliable and economical. We were subjected to numerous remarks, such as, "What is that thing? Why that could fit in my trunk as a spare!" or "Is that a toy?" Back then, it was the smallest vehicle the Wyomingites had ever seen. Today, Toyota is one of the most sought-after car brands in America.

Our trip to Salt Lake City was a success. It initiated many years of treatment for Stephen under the auspices of that wonderfully benevolent organisation, The Shriners. They provided Stephen with cost-free orthopaedic care for the next five years, and this would later continue at the Shriners hospital in Greenville, South Carolina.

Part of the mission of the hospitals was to include research into the conditions they treated and provide education to medical professionals. The Shriners Hospital aggressively entered structured research programs, and Stephen was enrolled in two streams of research: for the medical treatment of OI and for surgical intervention and 'rodding'.

In September 1967, Stephen, at seven years of age, had his first rod operation in his right leg. The doctors assured us that it was the best treatment that they could offer for Stephen's condition. Nevertheless, we were very worried and fearful of the pain that Stephen would have to endure.

I recall it was a wonderful distraction when our neighbour called on the phone and said, "Look out the window!"

I went to the front window and saw snow falling for the first time. It took my breath away. It was so beautiful and spectacular. Early in the morning, the trees were covered in sparkling frost like a thousand tiny diamonds in the sunlight. I had never seen such beauty before.

Rodding procedures were a relatively new surgical technique involving inserting a metal rod to support the long bones in the arms or legs. Under general anaesthesia, the tibia bone in Stephen's right leg was cut in several places, rotated and then 'threaded' onto a metal rod. The surgery required an incision long enough to expose the bone. The entire length of Stephen's right leg was marked with long surgical scars.

The aim of rodding was to control (and hopefully minimise) his repeated fractures and to correct the shape of his legs; his bones were becoming thinner and thinner and more curved. The rod would not necessarily prevent fractures; the bone may still fracture, but the rod would provide an internal support mechanism that could help keep the bone in alignment. Despite our fears, we were also hopeful it would strengthen Stephen's bones and maybe even allow him to walk freely.

For some children, the rodding surgery was a boon – it stabilised their bones and freed them from repeated fractures. Sadly, for Stephen, the severity of his OI hampered the success of the rodding and did not result in decreasing the rate of fractures.

Temporary analgesia in the form of a general anaesthetic provided relief during the operation itself, but the pain during recovery afterwards was intense. Knowing that there were more operations to come, for both thighs, we existed in a perpetual state of anxiety.

Every minute of every waking hour, we would wonder how our little boy was doing in hospital.

The Shriners Hospital in Salt Lake City had strict admission rules. Visiting hours were confined to 12-1 PM and 5-6 PM on Saturdays and Sundays. From our house, it was a drive of 365 miles (587.41 kilometres) each way to Salt Lake, and the time taken was dictated by the weather. In summer, the trip would take five hours or so; in winter, nine hours was not uncommon. We had to drive over South Pass, at an altitude of 7,412 feet. In winter following a snowfall, the high-altitude plains would be completely coated in white as far as the eye could see, and following the road required intense concentration.

When Stephen was an inpatient, we were only able to visit on weekends: two hours on Saturday and two hours on Sunday. During the rest of the week, our only contact with Stephen was via letters and postcards. We did our best to bolster his spirit with those, and we always included some words of encouragement.

In winter, we left immediately after the noon visiting hour on Sunday in order to be well on the road by nightfall at about 5 PM. Once night had fallen, the road was outlined by tall poles topped with reflecting 'cat's eyes', which went past as orange flashes for the entire trip home. Without these markers, it would have been impossible to stay on the snow-covered road. It is a wonder we never had an accident.

Our first hospital visit in wintertime taught us an invaluable lesson. Unfamiliar with the precautions to be taken to protect our house, we had turned off the gas heating system as we would not be home. On our return two days later, the water in the toilet bowl had frozen, our pet cat had licked a groove in the ice trying to get a drink, and the water in the goldfish bowl was frozen: and so were the goldfish!

We were extremely lucky the water pipes had not frozen and burst, a potentially expensive occurrence. We had not anticipated this as our Port Hedland days were only hot and hotter.

A few months after Stephen had his first rodding surgery, we were waiting in the airport in Salt Lake City, Utah, after a routine visit to the Shriners Hospital, Stephen said he wanted to get up onto a chair by the window to watch the airplanes on the runway. I was hesitant but also wanted him to do something he wanted to without me saying 'no' to everything. So, I let him. But he suddenly stepped off the back of the chair, fell down and broke his leg. My stomach turned over and I felt extremely sick.

A very lovely and compassionate elderly couple ran over to help me with Stephen. We took him back to the hospital. These nice people welcomed me to come back with them and stay at their house overnight and catch a plane back to Riverton the next day. I had never known such compassion from complete strangers. They gave me a lovely dinner and showed me to a guest room equipped with every need, just like a hotel room. I slept on beautiful clean sheets and had clean towels in the bathroom. They served me breakfast and gave me a ride to the airport to catch my plane. On the plane I started shaking and crying: not only for leaving Stephen behind in such unhappy circumstances, but also because I had not thought to ask this kind couple for their names.

When Ray was working in the laboratory at Lucky Mac, his workmates would often mention O.J. Simpson, who was a famous Gridiron footballer at the time. Ray would often interject in these conversations with a proud claim to fame and joke, "That's my brother!" Ray did not know O.J. was an Afro-American when he first started to allege that he was related to him. Thereafter, Ray became a keen follower of Gridiron. The Dallas Cowboys soon became his favourite team.

Americans, we found, were genuinely religious. We were constantly asked which church we attended, and the first response that came into my head was the Church of England. Subsequently, we were invited to join the Presbyterian church by Ray's boss. We thoroughly enjoyed it. We found that going to church offered pleasant fellowship. After church everyone got invited into people's homes for brunch consisting of all kinds of delicacies, fruit platters and amazing deserts. The social aspect was an immense help in adjusting to life in America. For Stephen, the seeds of faith were planted by the orderlies at the Shriners Children's Hospital. We were happy to see the comfort his faith gave him.

Sometimes it felt like we were in a non-English speaking country. Our countries were so far apart that some people were unsure what language we spoke. When we said we were from Australia, some people thought we were saying Austria. Since that time, travel and the internet have played a big part to in educating people and changing their perspective. Also, driving on the right-hand side of the road was a big change and required extra concentration.

I still remember the first time we encountered an Afro-American. We were driving around Riverton and had got lost. I looked over and noticed a Black man walking down the street. Thinking he would know the area, I naively approached him to ask where a certain street was. He instinctively stepped back and looked around to see if anyone was watching. He was very uneasy, but was able to quickly give us the directions we needed.

I realised later why he acted the way he did. There still existed backlash from the black-and-white racial inequality in America. A few years earlier, if a Black man talked to a white woman, he could be lynched by a secret society named the Ku Klux Klan. The Klan still exists in America today, albeit in a subdued manner, unlike its former glory days when it was active in persecuting Afro-Americans because of their colour.

Being Australians, we were treated like celebrities and always greeted with enthusiasm. The Americans saw us as a novelty and bombarded us with questions about Australia. When being introduced to strangers, they often asked us to say something in Australian. There was often a lot of confusion due to different names for different things. They called the evening meal 'dinner', we called it 'tea'; what we called 'holidays' they called 'vacation'; a 'car', they called 'automobile'; and what we called 'boot', they called a 'trunk'. Sometimes we would have conversations where no one knew what the other was talking about!

Ray's firm had given us a large turkey for Christmas, and with snow outside, the three of us had our first Christmas in America. We had turkey, salad, mashed potatoes, cooked yams with marshmallows, green beans and pecan pie for dessert – very different from our traditional 'prawns-on-the-beach' Christmas in Australia.

In the local newspaper, The Riverton Ranger, there was an article about Christmas and Santa. Children were invited to write to Santa regarding their Christmas present requests. Stephen carefully drafted a letter to Santa. The newspaper thought Stephen's letter was so nice that they printed it. What was unusual about his letter was that he informed Santa he had saved his very own money to help Santa purchase his toy, in case Santa could not afford it. His thoughtfulness for others was an enduring quality that continued into his adulthood.

Stephen still believed in Santa then, because Ray and I had heaped many presents under the Christmas tree with various titles – 'To Stephen from Santa', 'To Stephen from Santa Clause', 'To Stephen from Mr and Mrs S Clause', 'To Stephen from Father Christmas', 'To Stephen from St Nick', etc.

On Christmas morning, after Stevie had opened all his presents from Santa, he looked up at us and asked, "Well, what did you two give me?" We looked at each other and made an excuse that our presents for him were held up in the mail. We had to hurriedly buy more presents as soon as the stores opened after Christmas day.

Stephen found out that there was 'no Santa' from the other children when school resumed after the Christmas holidays. He did not let on to us, however, that he knew there was no Santa. So we did the same thing next Christmas – wrapping up his presents and labelling them as Mr and Mrs Clause! He later admitted that he knew Santa was not real but he hadn't told us so he could simply keep getting his presents from Santa! We later laughed and laughed at his subterfuge.

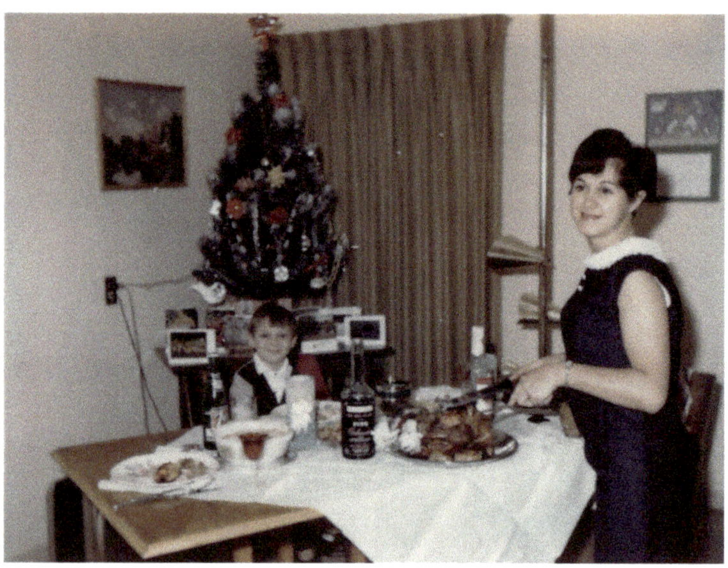

Our first Christmas in Riverton, Wyoming

6

Wyoming Days

Early 1968 we moved to a log cabin at 906 East Fremont, opposite the City Park, where every evening in summer there were displays of Indian tribal dancing by the local Shoshone Indians, each dancer wearing a full head dress. We were delighted, as it was very entertaining to watch. This same park was flooded in wintertime to serve as a skating rink for the locals. Needless to say, we never learned to skate.

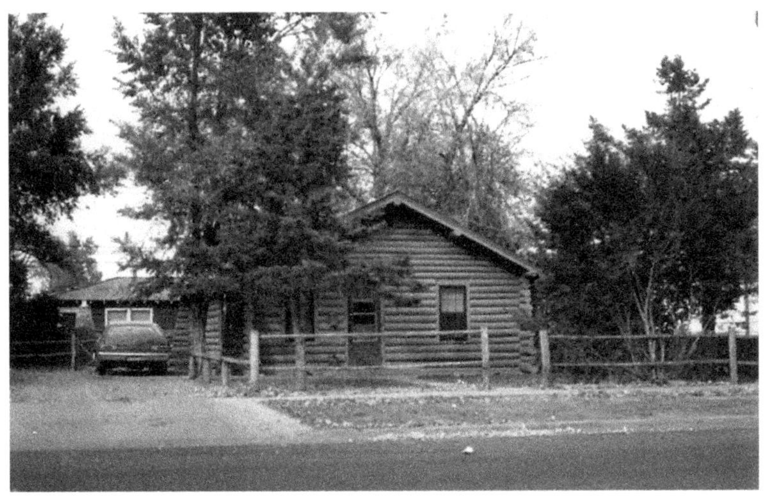

Our second house at 906 East Fremont, Riverton, Wyoming

Despite Stephen's physical struggles, he developed a quick sense of humour. He adjusted to school overnight, seamlessly taking on the 'class clown' role and entertaining his teachers and friends at every opportunity. One day, as I was walking up the corridor to his classroom when school for the day had ended, I came across his teacher outside the door trying to stifle her laughter. She looked at me and could hardly speak from laughing, and only said over and over, "Your son!" between guffaws.

Stephen's health had temporality stabilised, giving me the opportunity to broaden my mind and learn more about the American way. I enrolled to study at Central Wyoming College. I studied English Literature, Art, German, Psychology and World History. It opened up a whole new world for me from an educational point of view and introduced me to new friends. However, there were grim reminders of the war too. Every week, I would notice another young man's seat gone empty in the classroom as he would be drafted to fight in Vietnam. The Vietnam War was in full swing at this time. Every night the news broadcast nearly one hour of information about the latest battles, with footage from the frontlines. Ray, who was 28, had been sent a 'draft card' so that he could be called up for obligatory military training to go to Vietnam if required. The card was meant to be carried by him at all times, and to be shown on demand. Unfortunately, he mislaid it. We were not stressed because men with young children were usually conscripted last. However, the Vietnam War was always in the back of our minds.

One of my new friends in college was a fellow student whose husband had been killed in Vietnam by an eight-year-old sniper. He had been on a river boat patrolling the area when he was hit. She showed me his medals, photos and even a letter from Lyndon B Johnson, the President of America, thanking her for her husband's sacrifice.

There was going to be a moratorium in the town, and she asked me if I would like to attend with her to protest against the Vietnam War. It was a nonviolent event. There were hundreds of people carrying placards and shouting, "We don't want your dirty war." We marched up and down the streets with many of our younger college classmates. The town's entire police force was in attendance with their guns.

In 1968, two historical events happened. On April 4, Martin Luther King, aged 39, a noted clergyman and civil rights advocate, was fatally shot at the Lorraine Motel in Memphis, Tennessee. He was rushed to St. Joseph's Hospital, where later that evening he was pronounced dead. We were saddened when we saw his followers marching and singing 'We shall overcome' on the evening newscasts.

Then, on the evening of June 5, 1968, we saw live on television the assassination of Robert Francis (Bobby) Kennedy. His assassin was Sirhan Sirhan, who fired a .22 calibre bullet into his head at close range. Kennedy had just concluded a campaign speech at the Ambassador hotel in Los Angeles, California, and was about to depart for Chicago, the next stop on his campaign trail to be president.

A focal point of daily life for Stephen was the television. In the USA, there were many more channels and information available than what we had in rural Australia. The TV became an important source of education and entertainment for him, as physical activity could result in broken bones and pain. His formative childhood years were moulded by multiple creative interests. He became keenly interested in science, music, planes, cars, space and mathematics, and loved watching documentaries. His knowledge of world events was advanced far beyond the norm for a child his age.

Due to his inability to engage in physical sport or play, Stephen could only socialise with other kids through sedentary, age-appropriate activities. I would supply copious amounts of potato crisps, candies and coke whenever Stephen's friends came over to play with him. His little friends enjoyed a slower pace, playing with slot cars, and listening to music rather than running around vigorously, playing football, riding bikes and such. Stephen could not participate in those activities with them. Naturally, every now and then some friends would tire of the slower pace, and they would want to run around to release their pent-up energy. This meant playing with his friends was often suspended until they tired of the usual rough games and would come back for food and relaxed fun with Stephen.

In some ways, this was a valuable lesson for Stephen, he quickly adapted to being left in his own company. He never indulged the feelings of being lonely or bored, as do most children today despite all their toys, sports and nonstop entertainment. Stephen learned to entertain himself. He did not have a multitude of toys but kept himself highly amused with drawing on his Spirograph, sketching house plans, sports cars and aeroplanes as well as playing with his slot cars on his racetrack.

One fateful day Stephen asked me to take him to one of his school friend's house to play with the other boys. I was excited that he had the opportunity to enjoy the friendship of others. Not long after I dropped him off with the usual 'dos and don'ts' warnings for his safety, I got the dreaded phone call to quickly come back. My stomach turning over and over, I knew instinctively something was wrong. When I arrived, Stephen was crying in pain. It eventually emerged that the boy whose house it was did not believe Stephen's bones could break and had decided to callously test this theory by jumping on Stephen's leg while he sat on the floor.

I was ready to murder. I glared at this kid and said to his mother, "Keep him away from me or I will kill him." She looked at me horrified, and I went on, "Your little brat will go on as normal. Stephen has to deal with months of pain, plaster and wheelchairs."

We put Stephen into an ambulance and went to the hospital. As a result of this mean-spirited little horror, we were once again back to the all-too-familiar sequence of Emergency Rooms, X-rays, plasters and great physical pain for Stephen, while I watched on, heartbroken and sad for my dear boy. It was bad enough when Stephen's leg was broken accidently, but it was devastating when broken by a child thoughtlessly testing the boundaries.

In contrast to that horrible child, a little brother and sister who lived in the laneway behind our home would often visit to play with Stephen. One day they brought a beautiful Siamese kitten for Stephen, his first cat in America. We named her 'Coofa'.

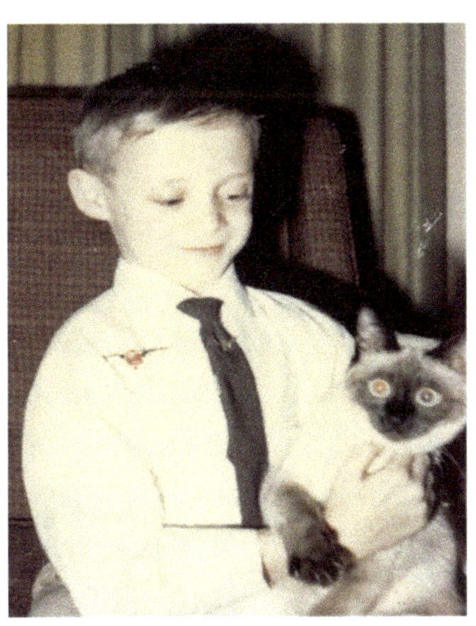

Stevie and Coofa the cat

We were in awe of the slow drawl that they conversed with during their playing with Stephen. They had the most amazing accent that would make us laugh. For example, it sounded like the following to us, and they paused in between each word:

"Iah'd laaked to hay-iv daaad laffin wain thayit muwel kaaked heem een th hayd [**sic**]."

Translation: "I would have liked to have died laughing, when that mule kicked him in the head."

This was how Stephen developed a lifelong ability to mimic different accents that would send us and everyone nearby into fits of laughter.

Stephen eventually began to develop his own American accent. Forever after, he would mimic the southern drawls and accents from other parts of the country and have everyone laughing hysterically. The more people laughed, the more he would mimic, while himself keeping a straight face.

These new friends of Stephen originally came from Shoshoni (so named after the Native Indian tribe) in Wyoming, a small western town north of Riverton, also located on the Wind River Indian Reservation. They were classic loveable hillbillies, with little formal education, simple clothes and strong accents. Their isolation had led them to be out of touch with modern culture. They were happy and content to be where they were in life, and despite being within easy reach of such majestic mountain scenery, the furthest they had travelled was to Casper, Wyoming, 120 miles south of Riverton. They were fascinated about us and Australia. They wanted to know all about Australia.

Likewise, we wanted to know all about the American West and its history. We learnt that we were residing in an area that had an infamously dramatic history.

With Stephen's increasingly limited mobility, recreation time was difficult to plan, but we made the best of what we could. We chose picnics as a source of entertainment. That way, Stephen could just sit in the car and we could spend hours driving to the chosen spot and back. We often drove 750 miles round-trip for a picnic. Stephen got to see most of America this way. We did not let his physical condition hamper his ability to do whatever he could. He greatly enjoyed sitting close to Ray and using one hand to steer on straight stretches of the road. Ray would be watching carefully, ready to grab the steering wheel if necessary.

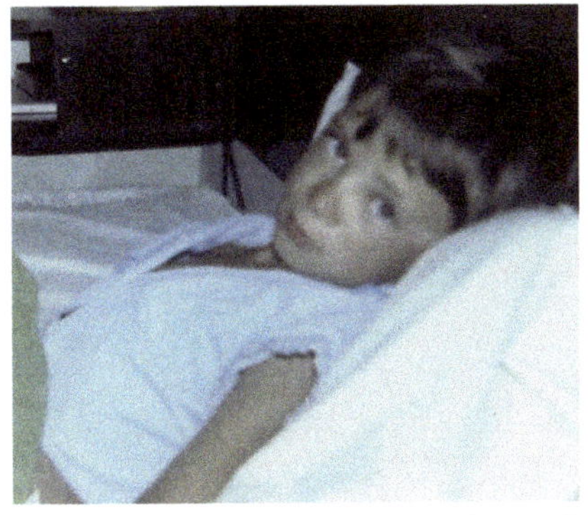

Stevie so tired after a day on the road

On many of our trips to Salt Lake City, we would take a rest stop at Fort Bridger, originally a fur trading post established in 1842. Later it became a supply depot for pioneers on the Oregon Trail. This further fed our desire to see more of the country, and we spent many hours in our little Toyota traversing highways and back roads in our quest for adventure.

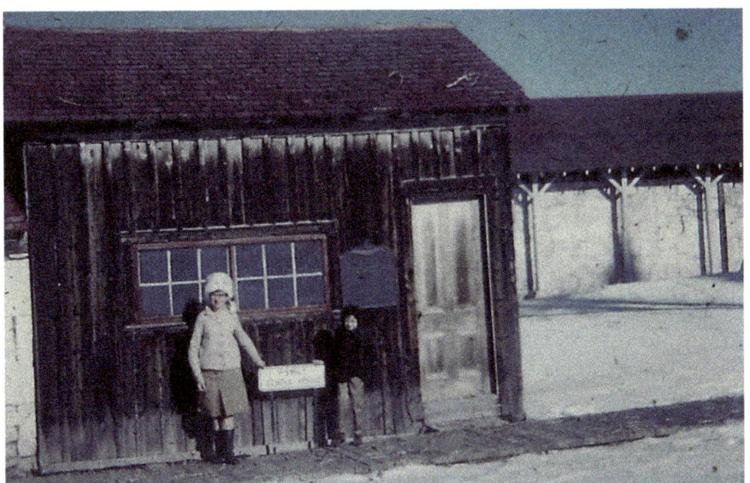

Me and Stephen at Fort Bridger

On one of our vacations, we drove through the Donner Pass on our way to Sacramento, California. We were stunned to learn that in 1846 a wagon train of pioneers travelled this route to hopefully establish a brighter future for themselves and their families. The group was snowbound for many months in what is now known as the Donner Pass. There were many deaths due to exhaustion, starvation, murder and adverse medical conditions while being trapped in the mountains. It is believed that those who lived through this terrible ordeal practiced cannibalism as the only means of survival.

Travelling expanded our and Stephen's knowledge of history in a highly effective manner, and was a far superior way for him to learn about the world as opposed to learning from textbooks. We travelled far and wide from our base in Riverton.

We visited Mount Rushmore in the black hills of South Dakota, and Custer's last stand at the battle of the Little Big Horn in Eastern Montana, the mining city of Butte Montana. At that time, the open pit at the Anaconda mine was the deepest hole in North America. One of our favourite picnic places was Grand Teton National park and the adjacent Yellowstone National Park. The sheer beauty of the snow-capped Tetons took our collective breaths away when we first stopped at the foothills. It was the first true mountain range that we had seen, and that memory is as clear as yesterday. Visits to Yellowstone were always fun and we explored the park from bottom to top. The herds of bison and antelope, together with hundreds of moose, were beyond our belief; we never dreamed such sights were commonplace.

Our first Fourth of July in Riverton was both exciting and sad. We were invited to a friend's house adjacent to the uranium mine, some 53 miles from Riverton, for a traditional Fourth of July picnic. It was a beautiful sunny day and the temperature rose to 100 degrees Fahrenheit at around noon. Shortly after, a bitterly cold wind came in from the Alaskan wilderness and the temperature dropped to 35 degrees F in just a few minutes. Meanwhile, Stephen, who had his right leg in a full cast, was enjoying the various festivities. Some children were exploding fireworks as part of the fun. One kid placed a cracker in a glass bottle and when the 'cherry bomb' exploded, the bottle shattered and a piece of glass entered Stephen's left leg, exposing the shin bone. Had the glass hit the right leg, the plaster cast would have protected him. This rapidly ended the celebrations for us. We hurried to the hospital, where the doctor closed the gaping cut with stiches.

One day, Stephen decided to leave home, for no apparent reason other than his natural curiosity to see the world. We said, "Okay, off you go." We watched him pack his teddy bear and his favourite slot cars into the tray of his trusty trike and peddle up the street in amusement. After passing a few houses, he turned around and headed back. He said he got hungry and came home for something to eat. Ray and I did not let him see us laughing.

In August 1968 a year after we moved to America, it was decided we would go on a vacation to New York to visit our American friends, the Hendricks. We had met Jim and LaVaughn Hendricks and their little family in Port Hedland, Australia, during Ray's time at the Mount Goldsworthy Iron ore project. They were now living in Jamestown, New York.

We were driving along a back road. The road was muddy from an earlier downpour, and we skidded into a ditch. Stephen's arm flung into the air as we skidded, and it hit the back of the front seat forcefully. Instinctively and quickly, I leaned over and with both hands straightened his arm, holding it in place while carefully climbing over to the back seat until we got to the closest hospital in Rawlins, 50 miles away. After his arm was X-rayed, the doctors told us that his arm had in fact been broken upon impact, but multiple chips and splinters luckily had fallen into place and his arm had been reset perfectly by me!

We continued our journey to Jamestown, stopping at the Chicago Shriners hospital where his arm was again X-rayed, and confirmation given that the bones were aligned and we could continue on our trip.

We arrived in Jamestown and were warmly welcomed by our friends whom we had not seen for two years. We reminisced about our life in Port Hedland and were delighted with baby Dove, our little 'Aussie'. We were taken on a tour around Lake Ontario, marvelling at Niagara Falls, on to Montreal and the 'Man and his World' exhibition, which was still open to the public then. We enjoyed camping in a large tent and having cook-outs. We travelled on to Quebec City and had a blast, until we had to reluctantly wrap up our Canadian adventure and return to Jamestown.

As a parting gesture, the Hendricks family threw us a farewell picnic featuring our first meal of Kentucky Fried Chicken. We were delighted with this feast; it featured again in many stops on our long trip back to Riverton.

One day, I rushed into Stephen's room to get him dressed for school and I trod on a coat hanger, fell and cracked the top of my tibia under the knee. Stephen could hardly walk due to his limited mobility and struggled to get to the phone to call his dad at the mine to tell him what had happened. Ray's boss asked his wife to take me to the hospital. I was to be in a cast for the next six weeks.

I had visits from our Pastor every day to keep my spirits up. I have remembered what he said to me then and found it true: "Good always comes out of bad, you will see."

Thereafter, whenever bad things happened to us, I would recall his saying and it would give me strength. Looking back, I have found that something good would always follow a bad event.

7

From Riverton to Marietta, Georgia to Huntsville, Alabama

In early June 1969 when Ray's job at the Lucky Mac Uranium Mine was finished, his boss threw us a farewell dinner at his house. Ray had packed all our belongings in the car ready to leave first thing in the morning for Marietta, Georgia, to stay with the Hendricks, who now lived there. I was still on crutches from the break to my leg. Before leaving, I went to the bathroom and as I moved to turn the light on, my crutch slipped out from under me and I fell down. I wrenched my knee and had to go to the hospital again.

Forced to stay in the hospital, I said a tearful goodbye to Ray and Stephen, who left as planned with all our possessions and our Siamese cat Coofa. They had an adventurous 1,550-mile or 2,500-kilometre trip. They stopped at Carlsbad, New Mexico, enquiring about a position at a uranium mine, where the cat got out the car. It took several mine employees and Ray about an hour to capture the cat. The management of the mine was not pleased, and Ray did not get the job. Continuing on, they stopped at every border state and took photos of Stevie under every welcome sign. They arrived at the Hendricks' place in Marietta, Georgia, about four days after setting out.

SANTA FE
TRAIL
Caravans from Missouri and
Kansas followed the old Trail to
Santa Fe from 1821 until the
coming of the railrod. The route
in New Mexico parallels U.S. 85
and U.S. 64 as far as Cimarron.

Road trip, 1969

welcome to
ARKANSAS

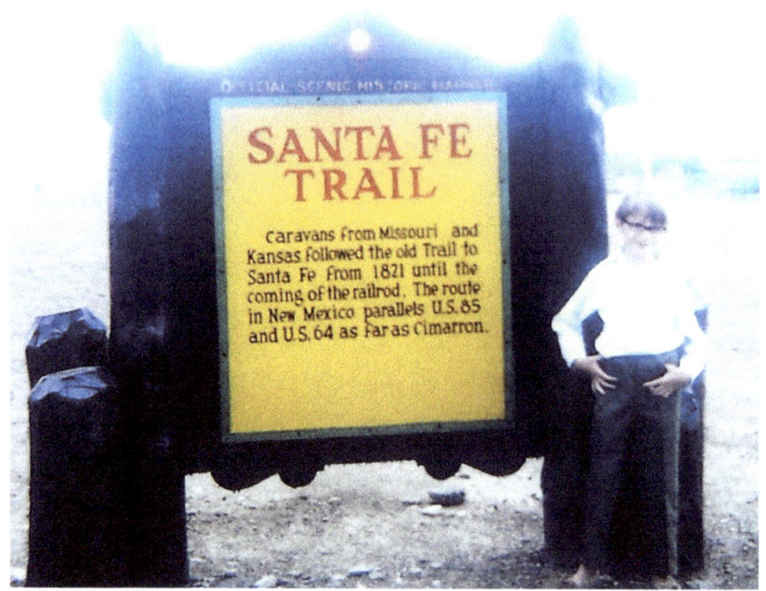

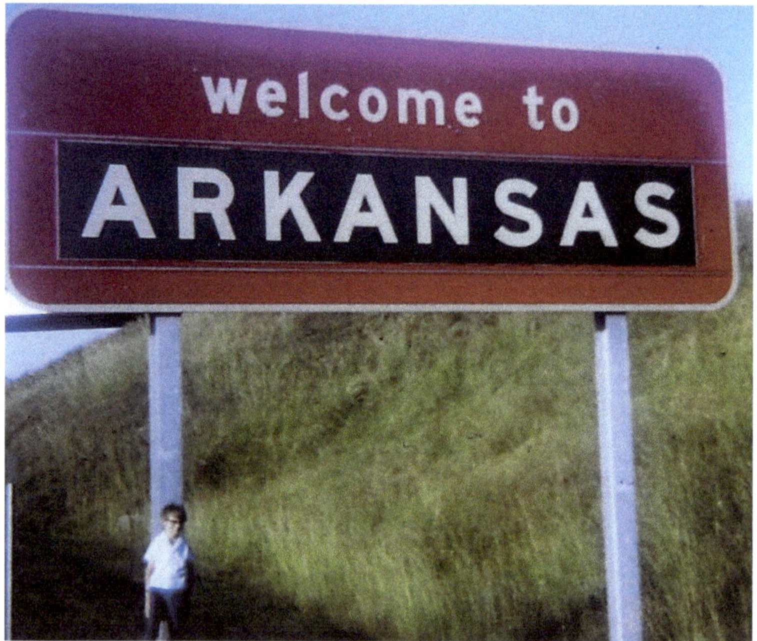

Road trip, 1969

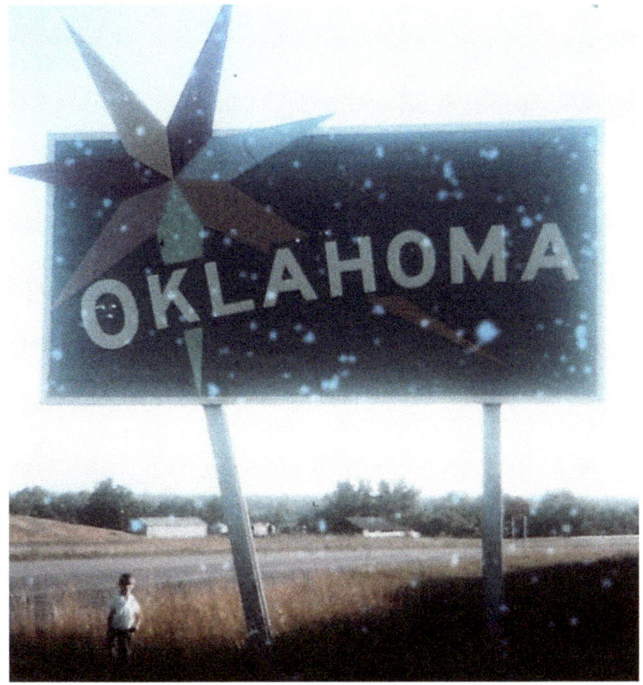

Road trip, 1969

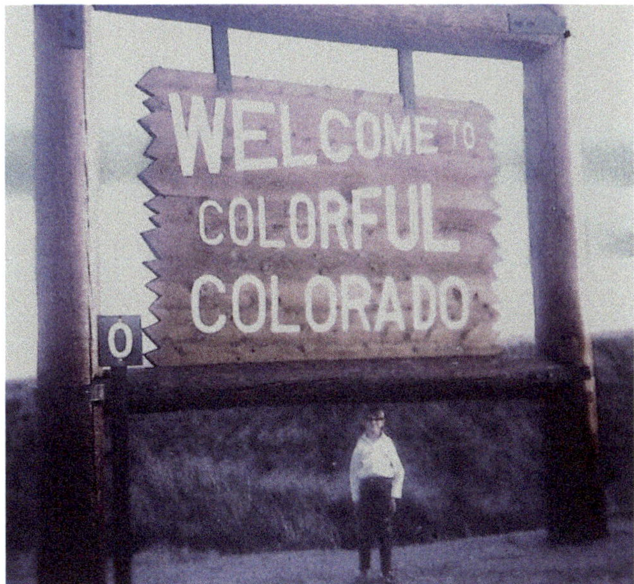

Road trip, 1969

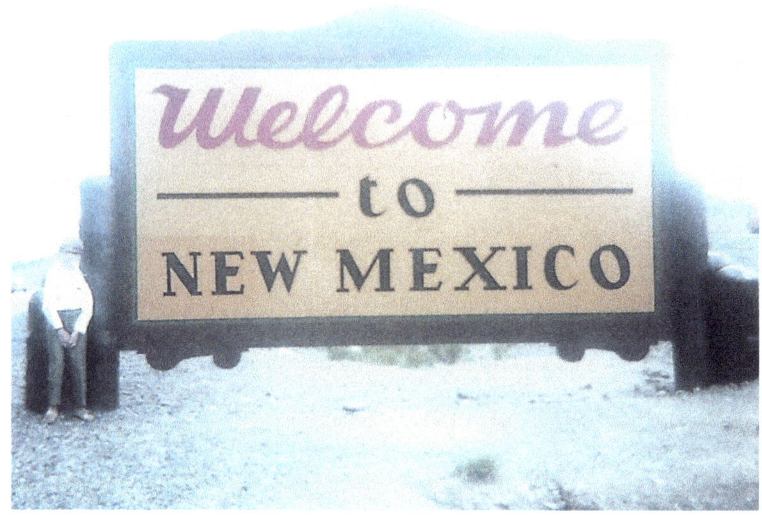

Road trip, 1969

I was released from hospital a week later, and I flew to Atlanta to be met by Ray and Stephen. Our friend's house was about twenty miles from the airport on Rebel Ridge Drive, Marietta, a very fitting address as neither Jim nor LaVaughn had ever surrendered to the Yankees and

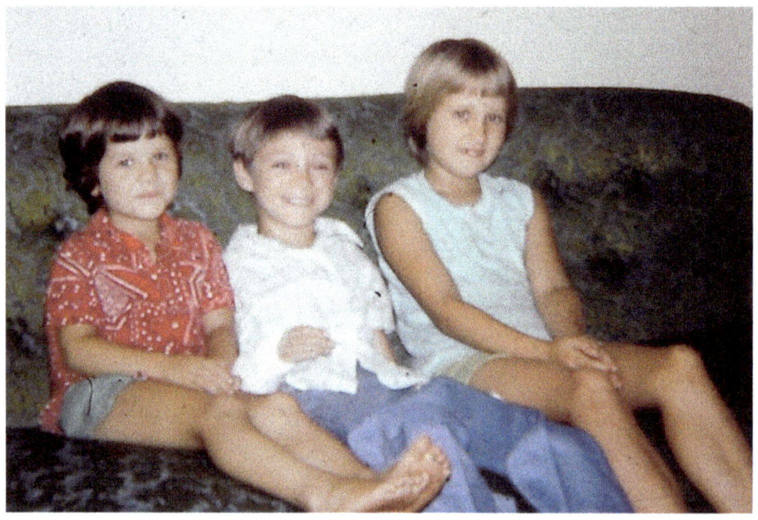

Stephen with Dove and Vicky when visiting the Hendricks, 1969

proudly flew the Rebel flag from their front porch. Stephen enjoyed the company of their little girls and perfected the southern accent daily.

At about this time, Ray noticed an advertisement in the Atlanta Journal - Constitution newspaper which simply stated 'Metallurgist wanted, please call' and gave an Alabama phone number. Ray called the number and was invited to Huntsville, 160 miles from Marietta, for an interview the following Monday. Ray decided the whole family would leave early on Monday morning and that he would buy a new suit for his interview.

We set off on Monday and arrived at Sears and Roebuck department store just after opening time. It was already quite hot, and our car was misbehaving; therefore, we could not turn the engine off. This model Toyota did not have air conditioning as the weather in Wyoming called more for heaters than air conditioning. Whilst Ray was looking for a suit in the store, Stephen and I remained in the car with the windows down and radio on, me recovering from my wrenched knee and Stephen's legs were too weak and painful to bear any weight. There were no suits his size and the sales lady indicated it would take three days to have one altered. But Ray needed it by one o'clock, some three hours hence, and after much hand wringing and threats, the suit was altered by 12:45 PM.

Ray presented for the interview at a huge factory where telephones were manufactured. After an hour-long interview, Ray was invited on a tour of the facility, which was just being fitted out with all the necessary equipment to make 5,000,000 telephones per year. Then he was asked to visit the cafeteria for a coffee.

Ray started to decline, saying that his wife and son were in the car with the engine running as the car was difficult to start. The manager interviewing Ray told him to bring his son in.

"Well, he can't walk," Ray said.

"In that case, bring your wife in," said the manager.

"She can't walk either." After a thoughtful pause, the manager said, "Tell you what. We will book you into a motel, meet for dinner, and get a babysitter for your son."

Later at the motel when the babysitter arrived, we caught a taxi to a very nice restaurant and met with the manager and his wife, and had a pre-dinner aperitif. But just as we were about to eat the main meal, I became sick and we had to leave.

Ray was sure that he wouldn't get the job now, but the manager simply said, "Let's meet in the morning, 10:00 AM. And call me if you can't get the car started. We have 38 chemical engineers at the factory and if they can't get it to start, then we are in big trouble."

At 9:30 the next morning, the car purred into life and Ray headed for the factory. The manager shook his hand and said, "Welcome aboard, you can start next Monday. It might pay to have your vehicle checked though!"

Never has so much gone wrong that has resulted in securing the imposing position of Senior Metallurgical Engineer in a large manufacturing facility – General Telephone and Electronics (GTE)!

We drove back to Marietta and celebrated our good fortune with the Hendricks before setting out on the next stage of our life's adventure. That weekend, we returned to Huntsville and immediately moved into a rented accommodation in the north of the city. This was a furnished two-storey house about five miles from the factory and close to Memorial Drive, which was the main road through Huntsville and a direct run to Ray's work. As this was a new facility, installation of the necessary equipment was still underway, and Ray was to be in charge of the heat treatment, punch press and electro-plating areas.

Meanwhile Stephen and I settled into our house and waited for our belongings to arrive. We had shipped them by truck from Wyoming and had kept them in storage in Marietta until we found work and somewhere to live. We made arrangements to forward the goods to the trucking depot in Decatur, Alabama, and when notified of their arrival, Ray and Stephen set out to bring home our well-travelled goods and chattels, knowing that it would take several to-and-fro trips over the 26-mile journey.

This meant passing by Redstone Arsenal, where huge space exploration rockets were assembled prior to being barged down the canal and on to Cape Kennedy in Florida.

As the day was quite warm, Ray took along a can of Colt 45 malt liquor beer, and when the car was loaded for the first trip home, Ray opened the beer, took a swig, then passed the can to Stephen.

The depot workers were appalled at this. Firstly, unbeknown to Ray, Decatur was in a 'dry' County where the consumption of alcohol was taboo. Secondly, Stephen, then aged nine, appeared to be significantly younger than the legal drinking age of 21 years. Thirdly, the alcohol content of Colt 45 in those days was 11.5% by volume, far stronger than the average alcohol content of 5.9 %. Needless to say, Ray deposited the remainder of the can's contents into a nearby drain and hurriedly proceeded to exit the premises.

On July 20, 1969, Stephen and I watched as Neil Armstrong and Buzz Aldrin landed on the moon, and Neil Armstrong spoke those famous words: "That's one small step for man, one giant leap for mankind." Stephen had followed each step of the exploration of space with keen interest and his excitement at the moon landing could hardly be contained.

Ray was away on a business trip for his new firm, and he immediately phoned us and asked Stephen if he had seen the moon landing.

“Yeah, Dad! Did you see it?”

“I sure did, Steve, and you will remember this piece of history for the rest of your life.”

Ray promised to take us on a visit to Redstone Arsenal when he returned, and the following weekend we made the first of many visits to the display area where these mighty rockets were installed. We were in awe at the size of these colossal machines. There was a model of the V2 from World War II, right through all generations of rockets up to and including the enormous Saturn V moon rocket, which was laid prone on the ground as it was too large to stand upright unsupported. All televised launchings over the prior years had been astutely watched, including the suspenseful Apollo 13 mission where the crew was endangered due to an Oxygen leak, forcing them to seek emergency refuge on the lunar landing module on the return journey to Earth. Now we stood in silent tribute to this enormous space exploration program, the men who had engineered it, the brave souls who were blasted into space and the heroes uncertain of their return.

On our next excursion, we took Stephen to the Alabama Space and Rocket Center in Huntsville, and there, by chance, Dr Wernher von Braun, a German Engineer, was giving a talk about the future of the space programme. We were thrilled to see the great man in person. He had designed the first American satellite Explorer I through to the Saturn 1 rocket for the Apollo 8 moon orbit mission in 1969.

Dr Wernher von Braun had willingly surrendered with his team to American forces after World War II. When von Braun and his brother escaped to Austria, they called out to an American private in broken English stating who they were and revealing that they were responsible for the design of the original V2 rockets in Germany. Prior to his surrender, von Braun had badly fractured his left arm and shoulder in a car accident. Stephen was amused to see a photo of von Braun's left arm in a cast from fingers to his shoulder, and felt an instant connection with von Braun.

Meanwhile, life went on. I enrolled Stephen into Colonial Hill Elementary School in Huntsville, Alabama, and with my record transcript of subjects from Central Wyoming College, I continued my studies at the University of Alabama.

Stephen began to listen more often to the radio. He heard the songs Let it be and Maxwell's Silver Hammer by the Beatles and asked me if I would buy the recordings. Stephen loved their music and developed an intense fondness for the band members, John, George, Paul and Ringo and their musical ingenuity. Listening to their music and singing along in harmony stirred his emotions and played a huge part in transporting him out of his world of pain. He collected every Beatles record, right from their early days to the ones produced after their split, when each band member went his own way.

About this time, on one unfortunate day, Stephen was standing on a padded lounge chair. He called out, "Look Mum, this is fun," and slid down the chair. On his second slide and before we could stop him, we heard the crack of his leg breaking. My poor innocent little child, I thought dejectedly. He could not enjoy the simplest of things without being in pain.

When he had been treated, I took Stephen to the Beatle movie Let It Be. I thought this would help take his mind off his recent mishap.

There was not a parking bay close to the movie theatre. I had to carry Stephen across the street and into the theatre. Can you imagine this sight? I am small of stature and Stephen's legs were hanging down past my knees as I carried him. The additional weight of his leg in the cast added to the difficulty. Still, I could always find strength to do the impossible whenever such an occasion arose.

We both enjoyed the movie with hot buttered popcorn, chocolate Hershey bars and iced Coke.

In the years to come, the Beatles music became essential in lifting Stephen's mood whenever he became depressed. He would play it at very high volume and sing his heart out.

One day while in a newsagent's, I noticed a magazine titled Redbook whose cover featured an article about a mother dealing with her son's Osteogenesis Imperfecta diagnosis. I quickly purchased the magazine, went home and began to read how this mother was raising a child with the same disability as Stephen. Tears welled up in my eyes. I felt enormous emotional support in knowing that I was not alone. Here was a mother and her son in a similar situation to me!

I immediately wrote a letter to Gemma Geisman, who had authored the article. Gemma quickly responded and gave me the contact details of other mothers with children with the same condition, all of whom had reached out to her the same way I had. Further, she provided the name of Dr Clive Solomons, a biochemist Ph.D. and Associate Professor of Paediatrics at the University of Colorado Medical Centre. Later, Dr Solomons confirmed that public reaction to the Redbook magazine article had enabled him to accelerate his research by 10 years, by providing subjects for an experimental bone treatment using magnesium oxide. He found that treatment with magnesium oxide lowers the pyrophosphate level and allows for a more normal action of calcium and phosphorous metabolism to cement together and form solid bone.

Through the dedicated work of Gemma Geisman, the nation-wide Osteogenesis Imperfecta Foundation was established in 1971, followed by a Chapter formed for the Huntsville area in order to further study the disease. I was excited that something was at last being done to understand and possibly find a cure for this terrible disorder.

Stephen's ongoing surgical and rehabilitation treatment was now being administered at the Shriners Hospital in Greenville, South Carolina, a distance of 312 miles (502 kilometres) from Huntsville – that's a six-hour drive with one rest stop. It seemed that we were never going to live close to a Shriners hospital! Many trips were made for Stephen's treatment. With each treatment, our hopes would soar. The slightest bit of good news about Stephen's health was immensely encouraging and made us happy.

On one occasion, Stephen came home after a long spell in hospital. We were full of enthusiasm, and took him on a trip to Myrtle Beach, South Carolina, for a holiday. It was a wonderful day, and my heart was bursting out of my chest with pride to see Stevie making a sand fort around himself with Ray. After an unforgettably happy day, we ate Kentucky Fried chicken and put a very sleepy and exhausted little boy to bed for a good night's sleep.

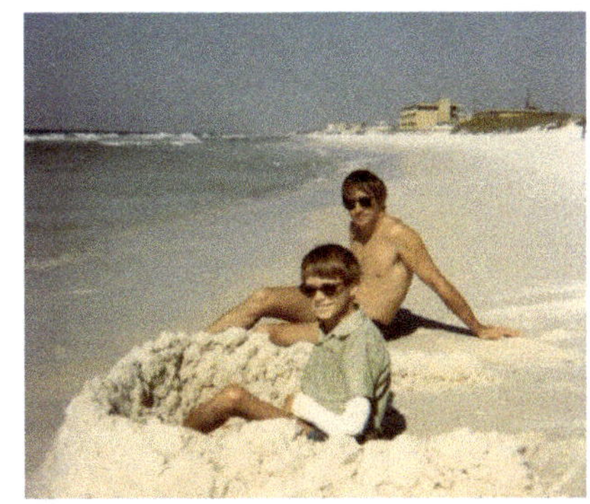

Ray and Stephen at Myrtle Beach, South Carolina

We also took him to NASA's Kennedy Space Centre at Cape Canaveral in Orlando, Florida. Stephen was so excited that his eyes were wide as saucers the whole time. We walked under Saturn V, the largest rocket ever flown. We touched a moon rock. We stood alongside the Atlantis space shuttle and re-lived the thrilling launch. It was a wonderful day.

In April 1970, for Stephen's tenth birthday we bought him a three-wheel 'granny' bike.

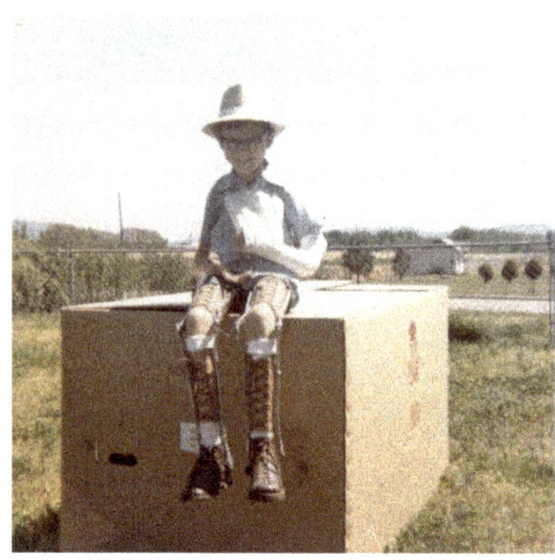
Stephen's bike arrives

We had by then become close friends with our neighbours, whose young son was a perfect playmate for Stephen. The two boys would ride their bikes around our quiet neighbourhood, having lots of fun. The three-wheeler was safe for Stephen, and he would ride at

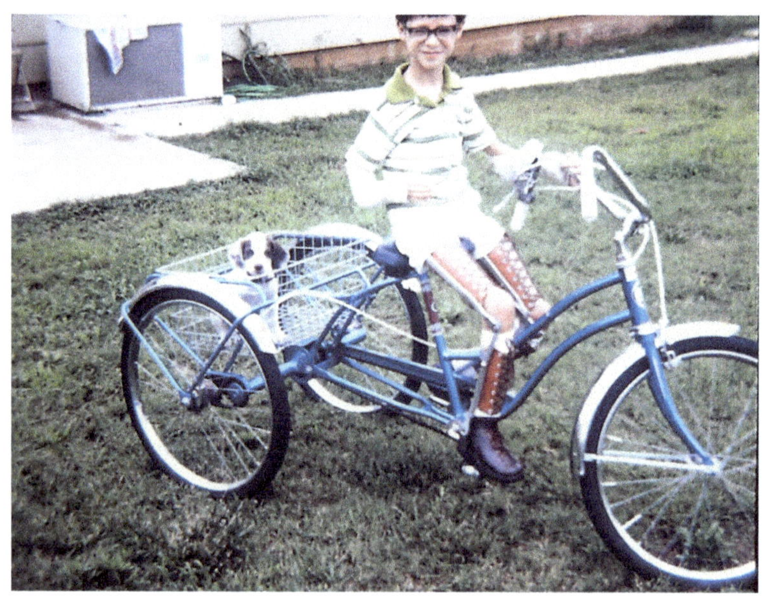
Stephen's new bike and his puppy, Butch

breakneck speed around the area while we stood and watched with hearts pounding, scared to death that something would go wrong and terribly injure Stephen. This was an extremely happy time for him, despite being encased in leg braces and having an arm in a plaster cast – this posed no hindrance whatsoever. The children of one of Ray's workmates also became regular visitors and joined in the frenzied activities.

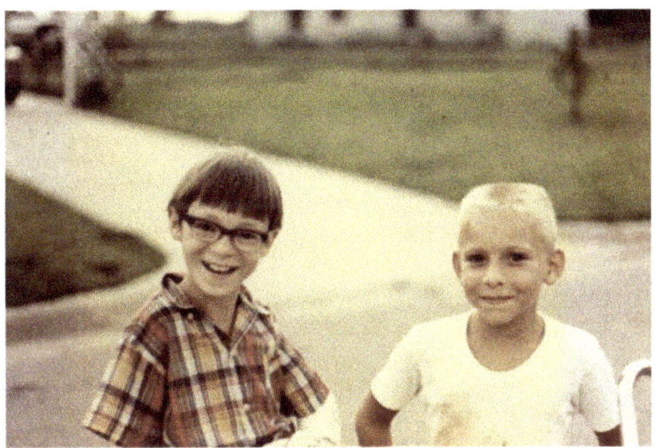

Stephen and his bike-riding buddy

Ray's work resulted in many social events with the management and employees. We were surprised that at the beginning and end of every gathering everyone sang 'Dixie'. It appeared to us that the south was still fighting the American Civil War from over 100 years ago. We would join in merrily, feeling very proud to be 'Southerners'.

Ray was progressing well at work and his metallurgical knowledge had expanded to material selection electroplating of various metals such as zinc, cadmium, copper, nickel and bright chromium, a feature of the public payphones of the day. He oversaw heat treatment to harden steels and became familiar with the many processes involved in making telephones. It was not long before he initiated several cost reduction strategies and improvements to some industry practices, which brought him to the attention of senior management. He was promoted to work directly under the General Manager of Engineering. This freed him from daily mundane workplace issues and allowed him to let his imagination run free over a wide range of departmental investigations.

Almost two years passed in this career broadening position as we further settled into the American way of life and became more financially secure.

8

A Visit from Ray's Mother, the Glasses Nana

By once-a-month phone calls to Australia, we learned that Ray's mother – or 'Glasses Nana' as Stephen called her because she wore glasses (Stevie had named my mother 'the talking Nana' for obvious reasons – was planning to sail on the Australis bound for Miami, via Sydney, Noumea, Fiji, Vancouver in Canada and then through the Panama Canal. We were excited by this news and decided to drive down to meet her ship when she arrived.

In due course she set sail from Fremantle in Western Australia. As befitting our family fortunes, however, at 3:30 PM on 22 October 1970 the ship caught fire near the coast of Noumea, New Caledonia! All 2,446 passengers were summoned to the boat deck while most of the 586 crew battled the inferno. The fire raged until 1:30 the following morning and the passengers stayed at their Abandon Ship lifeboat stations the whole time. The damage was extensive – the fire had gutted seven decks above the galley and buckled the dance floor of the ballroom. Water was waist-deep in the galley area after the fire was extinguished.

Temporary repairs were made so that the ship could continue to Suva, Fiji. Here it stayed for twelve days while undergoing further temporary repairs. The passengers were despatched by a variety of airlines to their intended destinations in America, Europe and beyond. This required great organising skills as Fiji was far from regularly serviced airline routes.

We were at home having our evening meal when the phone rang. Ray answered it. It was his mother.

He immediately asked, "Where are you?"

"Miami, Florida," said Glasses Nana.

A series of rapid-fire questions followed and the drama of the voyage was briefly discussed. The poor, tired woman had to seek help in operating the telephone and hurriedly told us she was being put upon a Greyhound bus and would arrive in Huntsville at 11:00 AM the following day. Our family got little sleep that night. The next day, the bus arrived on time and Glasses Nana emerged, clad in a flowery sarong, sandals and a large straw hat and clutching at her handbag.

We tried not to laugh at this sorry sight. All her belongings had been destroyed in the fire, and only her passport and some loose change had survived. Her travelling attire had been supplied by some kind airline staff as she was wearing only her nightdress and dressing gown when evacuated from the ship. As fate would have it, six months later, when returning to Australia, she caught the same ship home from Miami, but this time the journey was without incident.

The highlight of Glasses Nana's visit was the surprise trip to the Kentucky Derby on May 1, 1971, at Churchill Downs, Louisville, Kentucky. She had been present at a Melbourne Cup, the world-famous Australian classic, and we knew that seeing the Kentucky Derby had been a lifelong dream of hers – and mine too.

The trip was planned in great secrecy, and Nana's only instructions were to take comfortable shoes and pyjamas. We set off on a Friday afternoon and passed through Nashville, Tennessee, and Bowling Green, Kentucky, before arriving at Louisville just before dark. A frantic search for a motel led us to a decrepit flophouse on the outskirts of town, where we spent an uncomfortable night. Still the reason for our journey stayed secret.

Early next morning, on May 1, we had breakfast and headed to Churchill Downs where we finally revealed the purpose of our journey. Ray's mother stared in disbelief at the portals of the racetrack, visibly emotional.

When we entered the racecourse pushing Stephen in his wheelchair, two burly policemen asked us where we would like to go. We explained we had tickets to the infield and they promptly shepherded us trackside, then lifted Stephen in his wheelchair and guided all of us across the famous racetrack to the green grass of the centre. Their parting remark was, "Have a nice day."

Ray brought us four Mint Juleps, which consisted of crushed ice, equal parts water and sugar, a shot of Kentucky bourbon and sprigs of fresh mint. The glasses were inscribed with all the prior winners of the Kentucky Derby. This American traditional beverage was greedily devoured by us all on that hot day.

Just prior to the race, the crowd sang the traditional song 'My old Kentucky Home' made famous by songwriter Stephen Foster. There was not a dry eye among the 100,000 patrons present that day. This attendance record stood for many years and we believe most of them were beside us in the infield as we never saw any of the Kentucky Derby racers, except for a couple of Jockey caps in the far distance as they entered the final stretch.

The race was won by Canonero11, an Argentinean horse rated at no chance in the big race. It had been bought for little money and the connection had spent their last $5 on chaff for the horse on the eve of the race. The horse went on to win the Preakness stakes but failed in the final leg of the Triple Crown, finishing fifth.

Immediately after the race, we sat on the ground beside Stephen's wheelchair. Passers-by started putting banknotes into his now-empty mint julep glass. A short time later, unobserved by us, the glass and its bulging contents were stolen. Glasses Nana held on to her keepsake mint julep glass until she died in 1996.

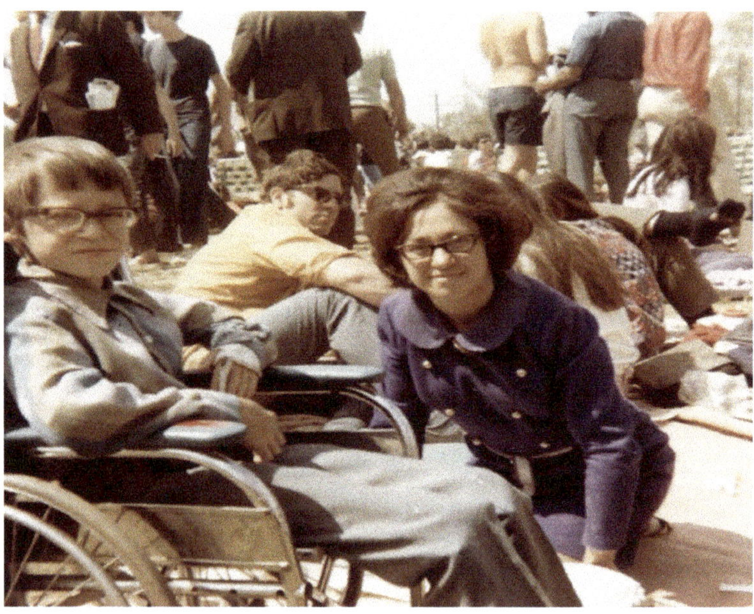

With Stephen at The Kentucky Derby, 1971

Unbelievingly, many years later in 2014, Ray and I revisited Churchill Downs as part of a river cruise on the American Queen and wandered into a bookshop looking for souvenirs. Immediately, I saw a book on a top shelf entitled Canonero11 – The Wonder horse. The book had been published only two months before our return visit and a copy now occupies a place of honour in our hearts and in our bookcase. We also excitedly purchased a small glass and a miniature bottle of Mint Julep complete with recipe as a souvenir for Stephen. We were in awe of the coincidences that brought this about. We had originally booked to cruise on the Mississippi River, which was flooded, and so we sailed the Ohio River instead.

Having been deeply moved by the racegoers singing 'My old Kentucky Home' at the Kentucky Derby, we decided to take a trip to White Springs, Florida, to see the Stephen Foster Folk Culture Center State Park, a distance of 378 miles or 609 km from Huntsville, Alabama. The 100-hectare park is a museum situated on the banks of the Sewanee River, about which he composed a song in 1851, 'Way down upon the Swanee River', a song that made the river famous. The building is a southern plantation style house, with enormous white columns at the front.

We learned a lot about his songs and plantation life through the glass displays portraying nostalgic scenes of life and living in that era. In one room stood a piano that he used to compose upon. In another room stood an old drop-front writing desk, where he had composed the ballad about slaves in a southern plantation. It began: 'Way Down upon de Peedee Ribber' which was later changed to Swanee River.

In 1935 Florida adopted 'My Old Kentucky Home' (also known as 'The Old Folks at Home') as the official state song. Seven years earlier, Kentucky had chosen Foster's 'My Old Kentucky Home' as its anthem. He's the only songwriter to have penned two state songs. It is ironic that he never visited Kentucky.

All the while intermittently through our tour, Stephen Foster's songs were played. 'Oh Susanna', a minstrel song, was his first big hit composed in 1848. It tells of an old man's journey from Alabama to

New Orleans: 'I come from Alabama with a banjo on my knee' was so moving that all of us had to hide our tears of emotion. Ray's mother favourite song was 'Beautiful Dreamer' published in 1864 after his death.

Stevie's love for music was further expanded. The best memory I have of this trip is seeing the pure joy of the whole experience in Stevie's face and Ray's mother's emotional reactions to the songs well known in her youth.

In 1855, in the remaining sad years of his life, Stephen Foster separated from his wife, and lost his parents and close friend. This, together with a dramatic decrease in his song productivity and mounting debts to his publishers, contributed to his alcoholism. In 1864, while living in a hotel in the Bowery, he contracted a fever and while probably drunk fell down and cut his neck. He was found lying in a pool of blood. In his wallet were just three pennies and a piece of paper that said 'Dear friends and gentle hearts'. He died three days later in hospital aged 37.

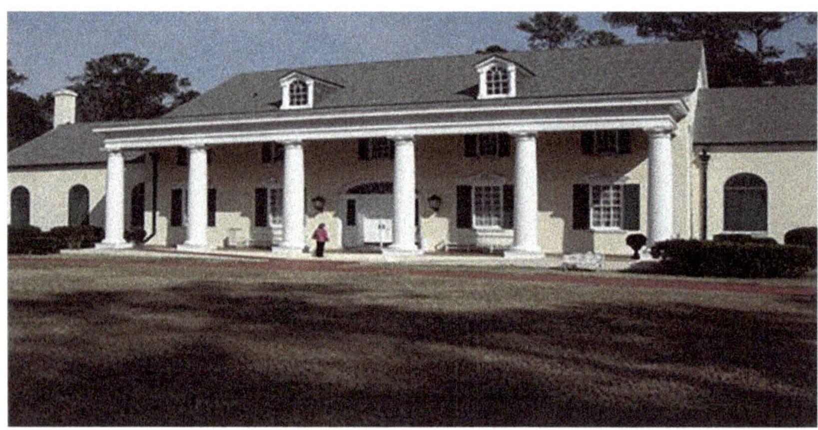

Stephen Foster museum

For our final adventure, on our way to Miami, we took Ray's mother to Tampa, Florida, to see the Busch Gardens prior to catching her ship back to Australia. Busch is the maker of the world-famous Budweiser beer and features the Clydesdale horses in its advertisements.

Busch Gardens was originally intended to attract people to the brewery. When it started in 1959, it featured only four employees and four parrots. It proved popular and in 1965 was expanded to allow the introduction of animals free to roam, while people were isolated in viewing areas. In effect, the animals roamed free and the people were caged. We spent several days visiting the park, which at that time was a ground-breaking establishment in the whole of the country. The introduction of a series of rollercoasters has kept the park updated and it welcomes millions of visitors each year. The gardens are spectacular and host millions of flowering plants. After

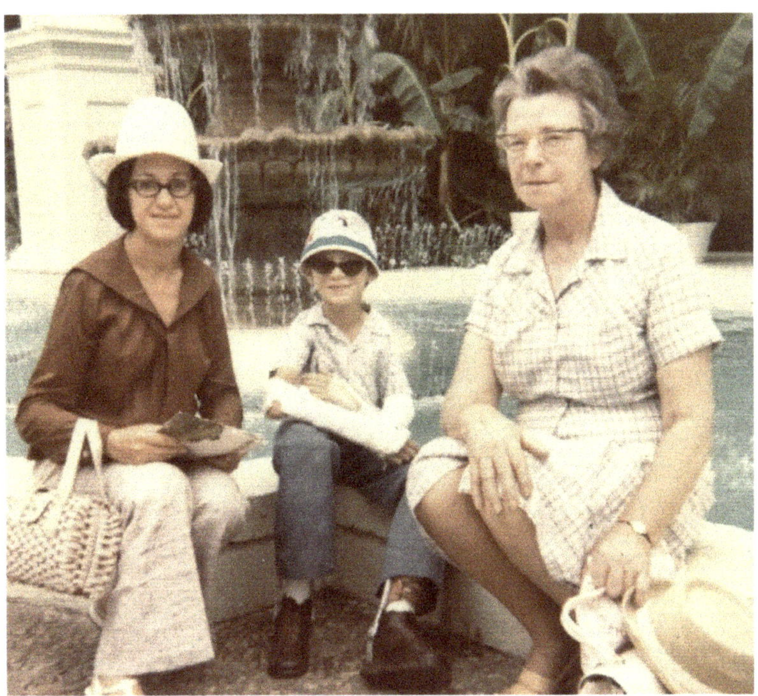

Me, Stephen and Glasses Nana at Busch Gardens, Florida

wearing ourselves out visiting most of the attractions at the park, we drove on to the port of Miami and bid Glasses Nana a tearful goodbye the next day.

One day soon after, Ray got a phone call at work. He answered in his usual manner, expecting it was a salesman calling. But the person on the other end said, "I hear you are a pretty good metallurgist and I want you to come and work for me."

Ray drew a sharp breath and asked, "What do you do?"

"I can't tell you that right now, but I'll tell you more when you pay a visit."

"Where are you?"

"I am in South Carolina," said the caller. "When can you come and see me?"

Ray thought quickly. "I have to go to the Shriners Hospital in Greenville in about six weeks' time. Will that work?"

"That's fine! I am a hundred or so miles south and I will give you directions!" The caller gave Ray his phone number and hung up, leaving Ray none the wiser about the offer than when the phone first rang.

Six weeks later, we drove to the Shriners Hospital in Greenville for Stephen's appointment as planned. Ray made the phone call to the unknown head-hunter and left us at the hospital while he drove to Elgin in South Carolina, a small town just outside Columbia, the state capital.

Here he met the Chief Engineer and Manager of a small manufacturing facility, obviously in pre-start-up mode. He was interviewed first by the Engineer, who placed two small metal objects on his desk and asked Ray to identify them.

Ray looked at them and replied, "They are left and right-hand stampings from a punch press."

"Right, when can you start?"

Ray asked what the facility was to manufacture, and he was told that it must remain confidential for the time being. Ray then asked about his salary.

"How much do you want?" the Engineer asked.

Ray named a figure several thousand dollars more than his current income.

"Good, now meet the others in the group."

A few more brief interviews took place, including a final one with the Chief Engineer focused on a start date. Ray was adamant that he must give four weeks' notice at the telephone plant. "Well, we will see you in four weeks then," was the response and the visit was concluded.

A slightly bewildered Ray drove back to Greenville, picked us up from the hospital and drove the five-hour trip back to Huntsville, Alabama.

A flurry of activity followed as we packed our belongings again! Ray completed work formalities while I terminated utilities. Stephen was excited for a new adventure, but sad to leave his bike-riding buddy as they had had so much fun together. Then our little family set out on the next chapter of our life's journey into the unknown.

9

Columbia, South Carolina

Ray arrived at his new workplace on the appointed day, while Stephen and I, from the sanctuary of a central motel, scoured the newspapers for a place to live. This resulted in the purchase of a brand-new house at 2921 Bancroft Road in Columbia, South Carolina, close to Interstate 26 heading for Greenville and State Route 521 heading for Elgin, some 30 minutes away.

The scope of Ray's work was then revealed: he would be manufacturing chainsaw chains for a branch of Homelite. The founders of the business had been engaged in this activity in north-western US and had decided to branch out and make the world's best chain for cutting the huge trees native to the north western States. Initially, there was much work involved in making the individual parts to extremely tight tolerances, and Ray spent many late hours in refining tooling to obtain these results. The finished product was indeed a world beater and was much in demand by the pros that worked in the logging industry. It was not long before Ray was subject to a performance review that praised his efforts and tagged him for future progress within the company.

Meanwhile, visits to the Shriners hospital, a mere 110 miles away in Greenville, continued on a regular basis. This was a straight shot up

Highway I26, then a branch off onto Route 385. The whole drive took about an hour and a half – a drastic change from the five-hour trips to Salt Lake City.

We slowly settled into our pretty, new house with its modern kitchen, double car garage, big open fireplace and, of all things, white carpeting. The open fireplace was a blessing in winter. As a means of quality control for the chainsaw chain, swamp oak trees were mounted in a sawhorse and a hydraulically powered unit sliced 1½ inch biscuits from the logs. After a required number of cuts, the chain was examined for wear, stretch and other engineering criteria, to ensure the product was within specification. Ray would eagerly gather up the sawn biscuits, resulting in the best roaring fires that kept our house toasty even in the coldest of winter nights.

On November 1, 1971, Stephen was admitted to the Shriners Hospital in Greenville SC. Doctors decided to put Stephen on magnesium oxide and to perform a 'rodding' operation on his left leg in December and re-rod his right leg in January, due to screws becoming loose took tremendous courage for him to have these operations so close together. He was very brave and an inspiration to the other patients in the hospital.

The hospital would keep us informed of Stephen's progress when we went to visit. However, on one occasion, Stephen underwent an operation unbeknown to us. We knew he was going to have surgery but had not known when. A day later the surgeon called and said they had done the surgery and the operation had gone well (even though it had not), and we sped off to the hospital immediately. Ray drove so fast that we were pulled over by a policeman. When we explained the situation, the policeman asked us to follow his vehicle and escorted us all the way to the hospital.

Stephen had expanding rods, which can lengthen as the bone grows, inserted in his legs in order to prevent the need for replacement.

Unfortunately, his bones were not strong enough to allow the rod to be 'anchored' at either end, and the rods just kept shifting, which created further problems.

We were only able to see our 11-year-old son during visiting hours, which were two hours on Sunday. We arrived five minutes late one visiting day after his surgery to find Stephen propped up on pillows with tears streaming down his face. "You're late!" he cried.

I could see he was in a lot of pain. I was looking around the room desperately trying to find something to say to take his mind off his discomfort when I noticed a boy in a full body cast from the neck down.

"It's not so bad, Stevie. Look at that poor little boy over there," I said. "All he can do is look at the ceiling all day."

Stephen looked at me sobbing. "Uh aah, sometimes they turn him over and he gets to look at the floor too."

An overwhelming rush of admiration came over me. I did not know whether to laugh or cry at Stephen having momentarily forgotten his

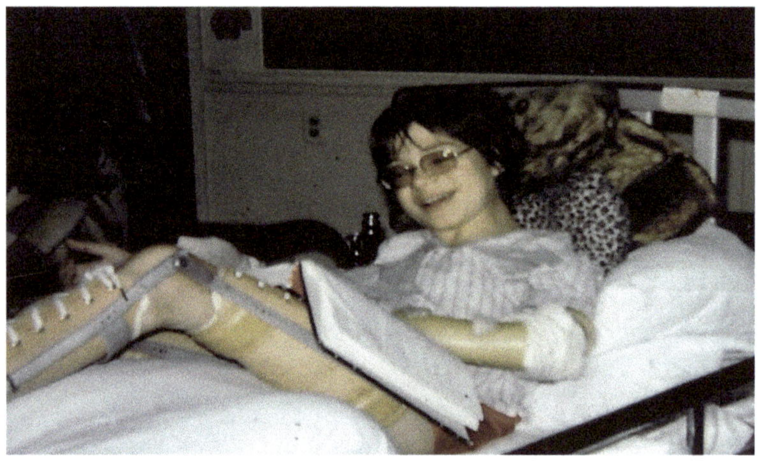

Happy waiting for surgery

own pain to observe his little friend's predicament. Many times, I have thought about Stephen and this day when I have needed to find courage for myself.

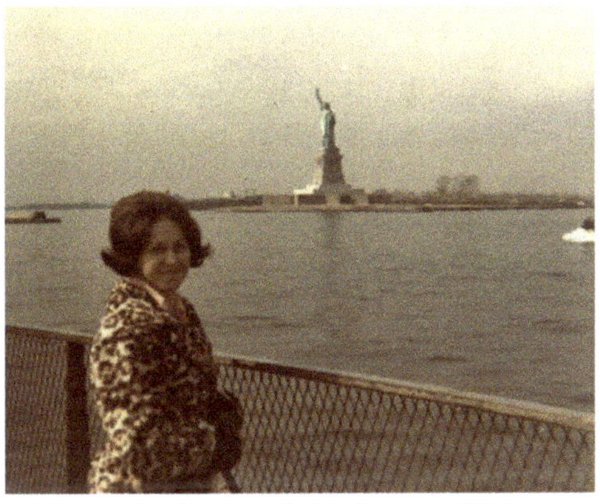

Me on the ferry and the Statue of Liberty

When Stephen was in hospital, and we knew he was safe I took the opportunity to go with Ray to New York and Boston for a few days on a business trip for his new job. The day before Ray went to work, we toured New York City, The Statue of Liberty and Ellis Island.

We went by ferry to the Statue of Liberty. We climbed the stairs inside to the top and looked out towards the Hudson River and New York City. We were clearly emotional at this experience, as have millions of people been, just at the sight of this grand statue.

We then proceeded to Ellis Island, which was a gateway for over 12 million immigrants to the United States from 1892 to 1954. It was amazing to see the huge interior of the large reception building. We could easily imagine thousands of immigrants milling around, being assessed by the officials and hopeful of a new and better life in their adopted land.

Stephen came home from the hospital in mid-March, after four and a half months. We went back and forth to Greenville all through 1972 for Stephen's numerous medical appointments.

One sunny day, while driving home from the hospital, Ray increased our speed as the roads were good and empty. The next minute, there was a blue flashing light complete with siren behind us. The Highway

Patrol policeman motioned for us to pull over. He walked up to Ray and informed him he had been driving over the speed limit of the speed he was doing, and asked him why he was speeding and in such a hurry. He then looked in the back of the car and saw Stephen with casts on both legs and one arm. Ray explained we had just picked up our son from hospital and we were trying to hurry home.

The officer stepped back and with a kind voice almost apologized for pulling us over, patted the car and said.

"Aah, I can see why you're speeding. This is a new car."

"Tell you what, (patting the car) just slow down a bit on the road."

Ray said meekly.

"Thank you very much Officer."

We were all afraid we were going to be fined and breathed a sigh of relief as we continued our way home.

The months passed and summer arrived. Trying to find ways to ease our boy's struggles, we considered investing in a swimming pool that would enable him to exercise without putting all his weight on his fragile legs. He was not very active anymore due to his condition, and a pool should allow him to have fun while he used his arms and legs in the water.

We were astute enough to get our local doctor to provide a script for a swimming pool. This foresight paid dividends later when it came to filing our tax returns.

We believed an above ground pool would be the best financial option, and we decided to partially sink the pool into the ground to make lifting Stephen in and out of the pool easier. Ray hired an earthmoving contractor to dig a large hole in our backyard to erect the pool. Ray shoveled a lot of sand around it to bring the ground level with the surroundings. We then placed a couple of paving slabs to allow entry without trailing sand into the pool. Next, we erected the safety fence and child proof gate, and, with a celebratory beer, started filling the pool with water via the garden hose. This operation took almost three days; the Fire Department would have done the job in ten minutes for a very modest fee.

It was a happy day when Stephen first entered the pool, supported by an inflated inner tube. The smile on his face was worth all the hard work to bring this to fruition. However, the pool did not bring any great improvement in Stephen's condition. Meanwhile, as hospitalizations continued with more plaster casts on his legs, Stephen spent fewer and fewer days in the pool. His arms encased in plaster were not a problem as the inflated tube kept them out of the water.

With the advent of winter, Ray made the decision to empty the pool in case heavy rains caused the pool to overflow. Ice was also a concern; therefore, a hose was used to siphon the water into an underground sewer connection. This operation took longer than the filling, but since it was unattended, time was not the issue.

When the first snowstorm arrived, we photographed the pool area. All that was visible was the fence and gate and a big black hole where the empty pool stood. A week or so later, we had a heavy rainstorm. Water was an inch deep on the ground and eventually ran down to the pool enclosure, causing the pool walls to collapse and its frame to bend. A disconsolate Ray pulled the remains from the hole and deposited the tangled mass out front, ready for roadside collection.

Sometime in the new year of 1973, we received a letter in the mail inviting us for a chat with a local I.R.S. representative. We were apprehensive as mail of this nature is seldom good news. We went along and were asked if we could prove our medical expenses, including our medical mileage. "What about this swimming pool deduction? Do you have a doctor's prescription for it? Can we come out and inspect it?"

Ray explained that the pool was now a casualty of winter, but we could provide a photo to prove it had existed. We promised to return with the kitchen calendar with all our hospital trips marked on it and the prescription with a covering note from our doctor.

We also provided the photo of the snow scene which prompted a sarcastic remark, "I suppose the expensive non-slip Italian tiles are under the snow?"

We assured him that was the case.

Several interviews later, we were given a clean bill of health in regard to our tax return, with a friendly suggestion not to claim for the cost of the sand required to fill in the hole left by our now defunct swimming pool. We were audited every year after that for the duration of our stay in America.

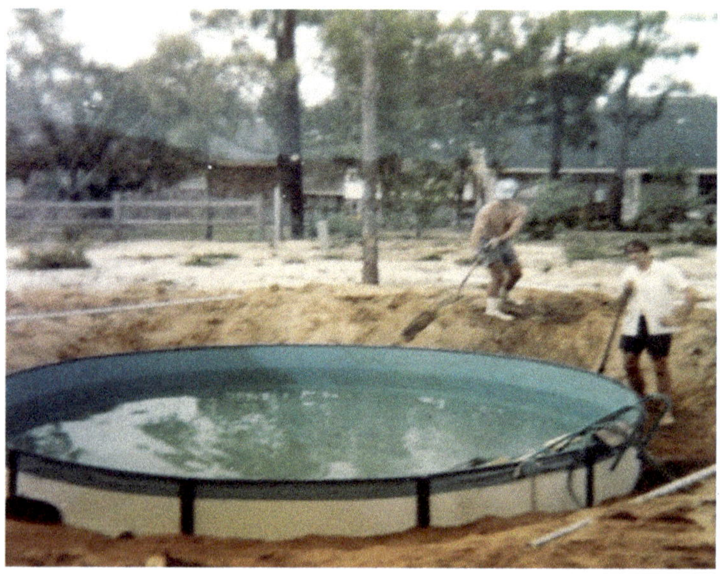

Building the above-ground pool

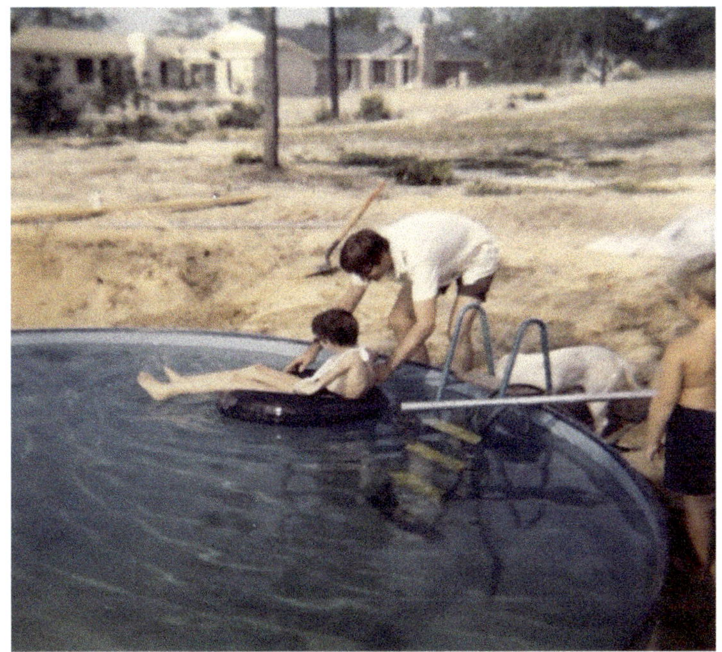

Stephen's first swim

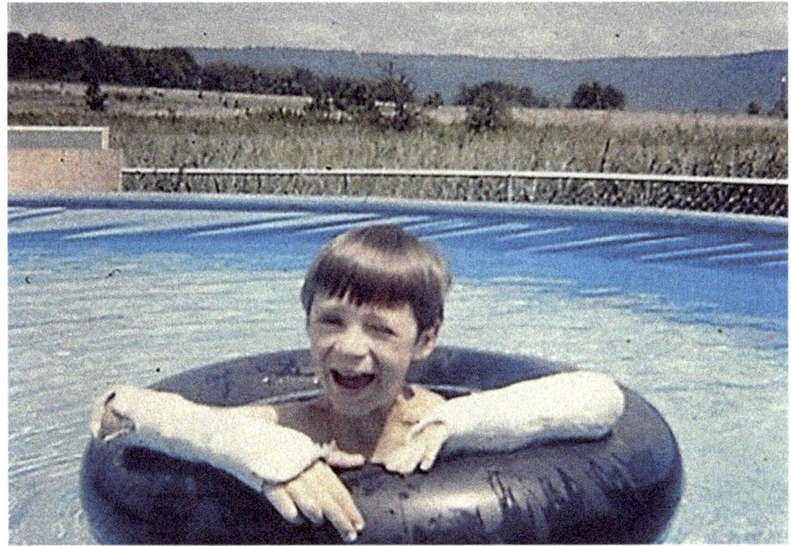

Happy Stephen could do a lot in his pool

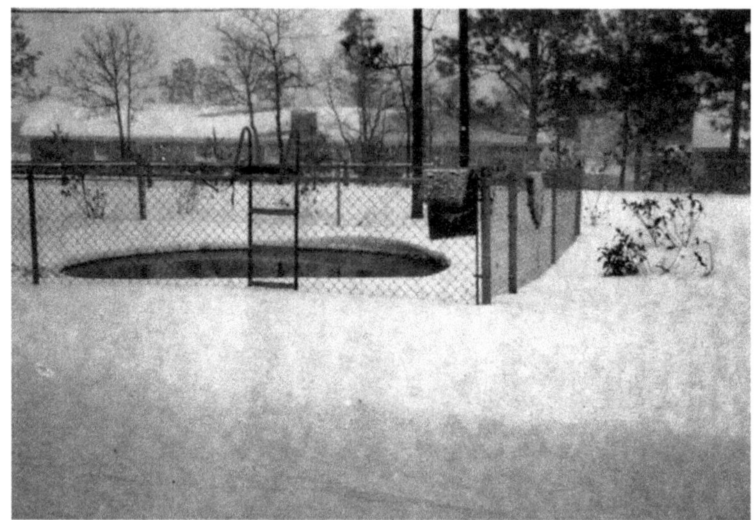

Snow brought the end of summer fun

When Stephen's health improved somewhat, he decided it was time to ride his beloved bike again. Every time the phone rang when Stephen was outside riding his bike or playing with his friends, I would shakily pick up the phone, anxious that someone may have bad news to tell me. Deep down, I knew I had to let him enjoy as many aspects as possible of normality even if it meant there would be an occasional price to pay.

One day, a little boy came running up the wooden ramp, which Ray had put in for easy access in and out of the house, yelling "Stephen!" My stomach turned over and my heart jumped up into my throat. The little boy went on to say:

"Stephen wants me to get Butch, his dog, to run alongside him on his bike."

I was instantly relieved, but held the little boy by the shoulders and yelled, "Don't ever come up to me saying 'Stephen!' like that!" The poor kid was shocked at my reaction, and I had to hastily explain that I thought something bad had happened to Stephen.

My mother, 'the Talking Nana', came to visit in the summer of 1973. She stayed for six months. It was the happiest I had ever seen her; she was excited about everything. One day she said to me that she wished she had been more like me as a mother and that she regretted how she had treated me as a child. I felt so sorry for her, standing there with tears in her eyes. I reassured her that it was quite all right, that I knew she loved me no matter her circumstances.

We took her all around Columbia showing her the many Southern mansions with their beautiful white columns, vast gardens and huge oak trees covered in hanging Spanish moss. She was in awe seeing these sights for the first time. South Carolina had been part of the South in the Civil War and had many places steeped in history. We showed her a big gun on display in a park nearby.

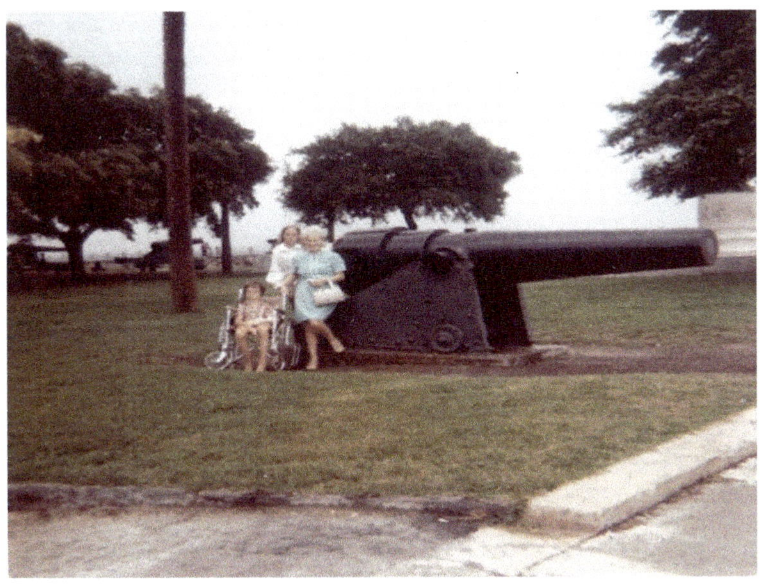

My mother, me and Stephen next to a Civil War gun on display

Another time, we drove one-and-a-half hours to Fort Sumter in Charleston, South Carolina, where the first shots of the Civil War were fired on April 12, 1861. On another trip, we took her to Florida to see Disney World, with Stephen in his wheelchair.

We celebrated that Christmas with the traditional turkey, gifted by Ray's company. My mother was thrilled with the experience of an American Christmas dinner. We sat down to a meal of roast Turkey, honey baked ham, baked potatoes, creamed spinach, candied yams, giblet gravy soaked up with buttermilk biscuits (scones) and corn bread. Of course, it was accompanied by some green salad and a dessert of pecan and apple pie with ice cream.

We reminisced about our traditional Christmas dinners when we were kids, having a baked chicken only once a year. My mother would add peas, beans, oven baked potatoes and pumpkin. Our dessert was always plum pudding cooked with threepences in it (a small silver coin manufactured in San Francisco at the time), topped with brandy, custard and cream. We would have lemon lime and soda to drink, also a once-a-year luxury.

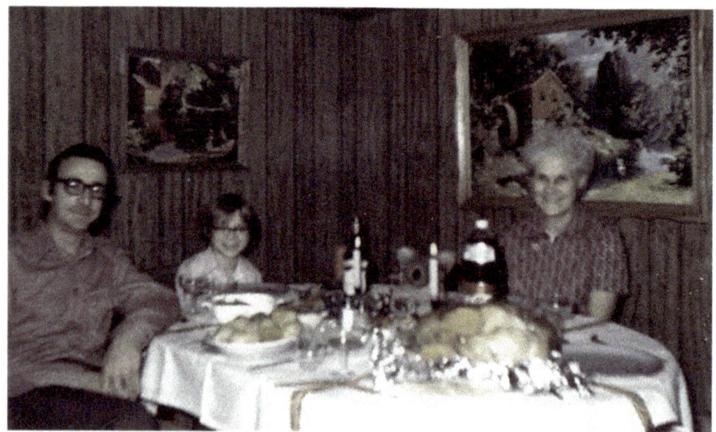

Christmas in Colombia with 'talking Nana', 1973

When the time came for my mother to catch her plane back to Australia from Los Angeles, we decided to drive across the country again to show her more scenery. Ray purchased a four-person tent and pegs, and we set off with the intention of camping at the numerous campgrounds of America along the way to save costs. At our first stop, Ray assembled the tent with the support poles turned the wrong way. Stephen, watching from his wheelchair, spoke up:

"Dad, the poles are round the wrong way. People will think we are Polish!"

Ray stood back, looked at the tent and agreed. He rotated the poles to the correct position, doubling the size of the tent, thanks to Stephen's observation!

We continued our journey along the interstate highways and gave my mother a glimpse of the big cities as they flashed past.

We eventually came to Wyoming, where we showed her the houses we had lived in, and proceeded to the plain at the base of the Teton Mountains. My mother was visibly impressed at the sight. Ray erected our tent, under Stephen's eagle eye, so that the mountains were framed in the tent's little window. We camped next to the Snake River, the filming location for that classic Western movie Shane. We always would watch reruns of that movie.

The four of us huddled together on that freezing night. My mother repeatedly pulled the blankets off us, and we were glad when daylight finally came. We hurried into the car. Ray started the engine, turned on the heat and we basked in the glorious warmth.

At Los Angeles Airport, we sadly bid my mother farewell. Tears flowed freely as she disappeared down the ramp to her plane.

In March of 1974, we received a letter from Ray's father containing an advertisement for a metallurgist to travel to Australia to conduct test-work on mineral sands, a common feature of Australian beaches. Ray half-heartedly responded to the advertisement and received a letter indicating that a principal of the company would be in Columbia shortly to interview him. The agent duly arrived and after a pleasant meal of cheese sandwiches, Ray was hired. We were excited at the prospect of returning to Australia, having been away for seven years.

PART 3: HOME AGAIN

STEPHEN AGE 14–17

10

Going Back to Australia

Ray had resigned from his position at Elgin in 1974 and embarked on a series of visits to Boston, Massachusetts, to work with a magnetic engineering company separating the various components of beach sands. The company had invented a radical new type of electro-magnet which proved remarkably accurate in separating materials according to their various magnetic properties, thereby producing pure zircon and 18 other products from ordinary looking sands. This activity required many commutes from Columbia to Boston. Ray always sat on the left-hand side of the aircraft and had remarkable views of Manhattan Island and the skyscrapers of New York on the way.

On one trip, while Stephen was recovering in hospital, I accompanied Ray to Boston. We took walking tours of the city and Cambridge, where Ray was working as a 'visiting scientist' in the magnet research department of the Massachusetts Institute of Technology (MIT). This laboratory is in demand from scientists all over the world and operates 24 hours a day and 365 days a year. He was conducting experiments on superconducting magnets, often working at 3:00 AM due to his power requirements, and when he tripped the super conducting magnet, it dimmed the lights of Boston. I felt very proud thinking back to the days when we were flat broke and living on potatoes with Ray attending night school.

Finally, in November 1974, Ray's work on the magnets was finished and we started the onerous task of preparing for our return to Australia.

We had decided to see some of the world on our journey home and undertook to call on various persons as a favour to our stateside friends. One of these stops was in London, England, to deliver some confidential papers for our friends in Boston.

We first flew from Columbia, South Carolina, to Boston, Massachusetts. Stephen was 14 years of age then, and through his schooling was well-versed in American history. He had learnt about the American war of Independence, and so we took him on a tour of the city following the Freedom Trail. This was a walking trail outlined by red bricks sunk into the sidewalk or by red paint where bricks are not practical. Stephen was well rugged up against the December cold but the cobblestone sidewalks were not exactly smooth sailing for him and not much fun for Ray pushing him either, as his hands blistered from holding the handles tight on Stephen's wheelchair.

At each historical site there is a marker, giving details of why the site is famous. We started at Boston Common and passed the Old Corner Bookstore, Faneuil Hall and went all the way to Paul Revere House. Stephen knew well the story of Paul Revere and his famous midnight ride to Lexington to warn the American patriots John Hancock and Samuel Adams of a British invasion.

Then it was time for us to head for the airport and fly to the JFK Airport in New York. While we were unloading our luggage from the taxi at Boston's Logan airport, Ray noticed his briefcase was

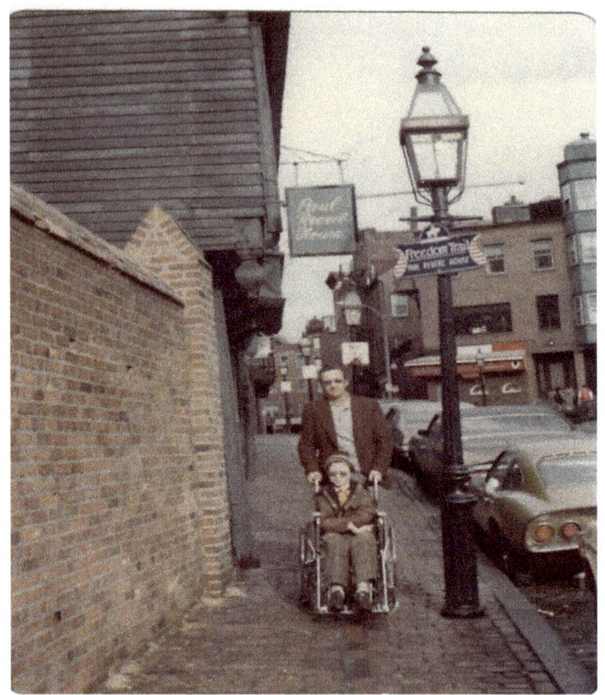

Ray and Stephen outside Paul Revere House in Boston, Massachusetts

missing. Panic! The briefcase contained our tickets, passports, traveller's checks and the confidential package from a business associate for London delivery. Luckily, we remembered the name of the taxi company, and a frantic phone call resulted in an all-cabs call to their taxis asking them to check for our briefcase. Thankfully, within 20 or so minutes, the briefcase was safe in our hands again and the taxi driver was amply rewarded.

We stayed for two nights in New York and managed to visit the Empire State building and took the Staten Island ferry to give Stephen a close-up view of the Statue of Liberty. We showed Stephen the Metropolitan Opera at Lincoln Centre, where Ray and I had previously seen the opera Carmen. Stephen was impressed with the architecture and skyscrapers for which New York is famous.

We made our way to JFK on December 9, 1974, and flew to London, England. A phone call to our intended contact yielded directions to an office alongside a bomb site, which to us was very confusing. A taxi driver delivered us to the address where we were amazed to see a bomb crater! This in 1974! We found it amazing that a bomb crater was still in suburban London 29 years after World War II had ended.

With our mission to deliver the parcel completed, the grateful recipient treated us to a fine meal at a swanky French restaurant, partly in appreciation and partly, I now think, to emphasize our ignorance of French cuisine. After dinner we went back to the Central Park Hotel and would have frozen to death if it hadn't been for 'doonas' for our bed covers.

Since Stephen was by now a fanatical Beatles fan, we were obliged to rent a car and drive to the Crosswalk at Abbey Road, made famous by the photograph of the Beatles crossing the road, with bare-footed Paul McCartney causing wild rumours of his demise. Then we went on to Penny Lane, after receiving directions from an elderly man who had a broad, almost incomprehensible accent. Stephen was ecstatic. All the way back to our London hotel, he could speak of nothing other than the Beatles and his joy at visiting these 'holy' places.

The weather was damp and gloomy, limiting our sightseeing to driving around London. We drove across Tower Bridge and shortly after saw a ship pass through. We saw Piccadilly Circus, Trafalgar Square and the street views of Buckingham Palace and the Houses of Parliament. We then proceeded to Stratford upon Avon, where we pushed Stephen around in his wheelchair to Shakespeare's birthplace and Anne Hathaway's Cottage, the childhood home of Shakespeare's wife. Having done many assignments for my English teacher in Wyoming, who was well read with Shakespeare's works, I found this to be the highlight of the visit. It also exposed Stephen to some great English literature.

The next day, on December 13, we flew to historic Vienna to fulfil my dream of seeing the famous Lipizzaner horses at the Spanish Riding School in the heart of the city. These famous horses had been rescued from the advancing Russian army in Czechoslovakia in May 1945 under the leadership of General George Patton. There was great fear among the defeated nations that the horses would be slaughtered for food supplies for the Russian army, so friend and foe alike transferred the horses to safety to Austria, where they performed twice for an enthralled General Patton and several other times for regular victorious troops. After spending the best part of a day watching these horses perform, I yielded to Ray's request to retire to our hotel and prepare for our visit to Schonbrunn Palace the next morning.

We left on our escorted tour on a chilly, overcast day and arrived at this magnificent structure renowned throughout history. We were amazed at the size of the rooms, the splendour of the furnishings, the paintings, chandeliers, the ceilings and the parquet flooring, and how the royalty lived in the olden days, particularly in the court of Maria Teresa and the Russian Emperors.

We were delighted at the huge painting in which young Mozart is featured, supposedly after asking Marie Antoinette to marry him, during his visit with his father and sister in October 1762. Had he done so when he had grown up, there is no doubt the course of history would have changed, and Marie Antoinette would probably have kept her head! We briefly visited the beautiful gardens, not at their peak in December, before returning to our hotel, aware we had trodden in the footsteps of many notable figures of history.

Next morning, we hired a small car and bravely set out on an Autobahn on our way to Salzburg, the birthplace of Mozart. It was a cold day, and we barrelled along until we arrived at the border. Ray went to the trunk to fetch his briefcase to get our passports and found that he could not open it. No amount of jiggling the keys or trying to pry the trunk open seemed to do any good, so we asked the border guards to ring for a mechanic. While we waited for him to arrive, we headed to the border restaurant and drank hot chocolate in the nice warm surroundings.

An eternity later, the mechanic appeared but with an air of having had better things to do this close to Christmas. He endeavoured to open the trunk without success, becoming visibly displeased as time went by. Ray, who was standing beside the car, placed the mechanic's large screwdriver in the gap between the mudguard and the trunk lid, applied some leverage and the lid popped open. The mechanic glared at Ray, muttered something that sounded like 'Dumme Auslander', accepted the banknotes proffered, gathered his tools and drove off with his tyres squealing.

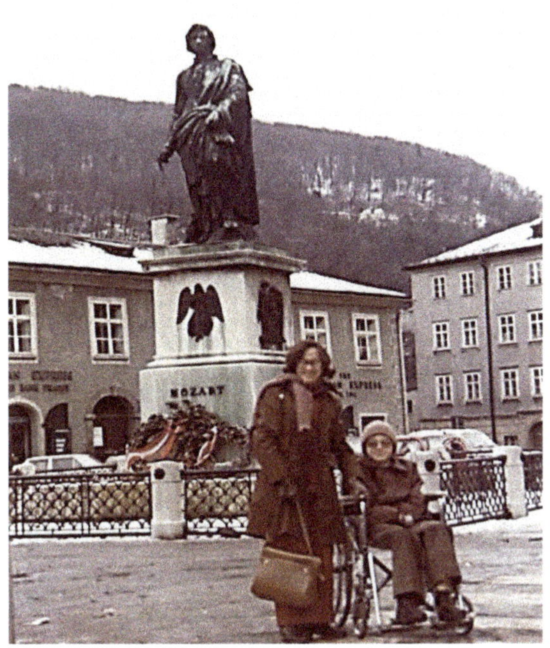

Me, Stephen, and Mozart's statue

Formalities at the border were quickly concluded; we resumed out travels and arrived at our hotel in the late afternoon. Stephen's passion for music was bubbling to the surface again as he contemplated visiting the birthplace of Mozart. This was especially evident the next day, when we visited the house where Mozart was born and viewed some of the instruments that he had composed upon.

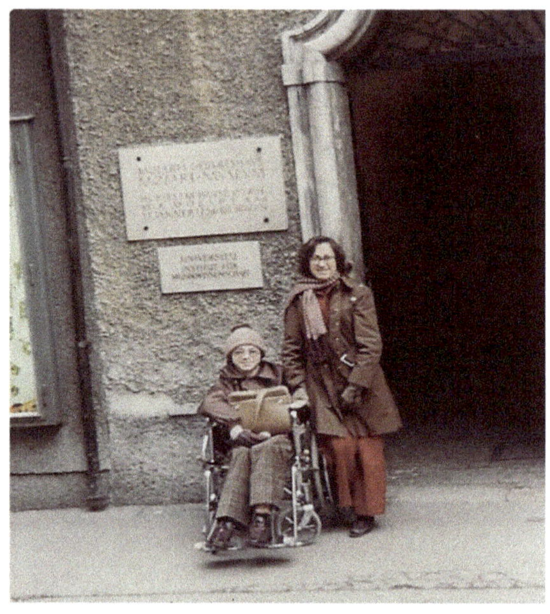

Me and Stephen at Mozart Museum

We spent several hours visiting the various rooms amid a hushed atmosphere, as all the tourists present seemed to be aware of the great achievements in this household. Stephen was intrigued with Mozart's harpsichord that he had played when he was only three years old. There were original letters written by the family, photos and all kinds of memorabilia.

We continued to explore the narrow streets of Salzburg, posing for photographs at places associated with Mozart and seeing the Archbishop's castle high on the mountain not far from the city. We spent the next day, December 18, just as tourists winding our way over cobbled streets enjoying the Christmas atmosphere, all the while trying to pick the smoothest passage for Stephen in his wheelchair.

An early wake-up call next morning had us hurrying out of bed, having breakfast and taking a taxi to the airport for our flight to India. We were flying with Air India on this leg of the trip and were delighted to have the crew in their saris hovering over us, constantly asking if we needed anything. They were aware of Stephen's left arm being in a plaster cast and we had removed his leg braces to make him more comfortable. He loved every minute of flying in an airplane, especially the take off and landings.

We made a stop in Beirut but did not leave our seats as the stop was only a short one. We were appalled at the number of uniformed men armed with automatic weapons that we could see out of our seat window. There was considerable unrest in Lebanon at that time, due to various factions trying to align with external powers in order to become the predominant governing body. These divisive factions ultimately led to Lebanon being engaged in a civil war that lasted 15 years and resulted in approximately 240,000 casualties.

Next stop was Bombay, now Mumbai. Here we had to deplane to go through Customs and Immigration. The terminal building was huge and packed with hundreds of people, all trying to get to the few Immigration officers on duty. There was no way we could negotiate the crowd while pushing the wheelchair, so we sat down on stools at one edge of the vast hall and waited for the crowd to thin out. This did not happen due to new planes landing. Luckily, a hostess from our flight noticed us, and after listening to our predicament, she ushered us through the Crew immigration station and on to our connecting plane, which was preparing to take off. We saw very little of Mumbai, and had she not intervened, I think we would still be sitting in that hot, steamy Immigration Hall.

We flew on to our final stop in India, the City of Calcutta, now Kolkata, to meet up with Ramesh Roy, the brother of our good friend from Huntsville, Alabama, Upendra Roy. Once again, we were crushed and jostled as we made our way through Immigration, baggage collection and Customs. Our passports duly stamped, we made our way outside to a taxi rank. The heat was stifling, and we were besieged by an army of children, hands extended and seeking money, or 'backsheesh' as we knew it. Hundreds of little urchins were crowding around anyone who had the appearance of a tourist, and Stephen's wheelchair was like a magnet to them.

We eventually arrived at The Grand Oberoi Hotel, where we were met by turbaned doormen and bellboys, and ushered through registration with many bows and signs of deference and whisked up to our palatial room. There were servants everywhere. It appears that this was the custom at the time. One servant was assigned to our room and he stayed with us until we went to bed.

After our evening meal of a spicy curry, we retired for the night, only to wake up early in the morning, due probably to jet lag and the stress of travelling. It was eerily quiet, and Ray and I stood at the window of our sixth-floor room and gazed at the scenery lit by the rising sun. Shortly afterwards, people and trucks, cars, and trams appeared on the street and the noise increased until it was a constant dull roar, perforated by the sounds of many horns from the traffic below. Soon the street was bustling with pedestrians and traffic all vying for passage to their various destinations.

We breakfasted and set out with Stephen in his wheelchair with Ramesh Roy as our guide. Ramesh was happy to meet us and had received a letter from his brother Upendra, notifying him of our arrival at the hotel. He arrived shortly after breakfast and was now pleased to escort us around a small portion of this massive city.

Once again, Stephen's wheelchair was the centre of attention and we soon had a crowd of children following on behind. Eventually, we ducked into a souvenir shop and the crowd disappeared into the river of humanity surging down the street. We spent a pleasant day with Ramesh and invited him to join us for our evening meal at the hotel. Ramesh was a great help in deciphering the menu, and the ensuing meal was much better than had we hidden in our room and ordered a hamburger.

Finally, it was time to continue our journey homeward. We had purchased economy class seats on all our flights home, but when the British Airways crew saw Stephen's plaster and braces, we were upgraded to Business Class on the 747 Jumbo. Aeroplanes had always been of great interest to Stephen, ever since he was a child. Now, here he was in business class on the mightiest planes of them all, the Boeing 747. He was beside himself as we carried him – Ray holding him under the arms and I supporting his legs and walking backwards – up the staircase to our luxury upgraded seats. We settled in and had a growing sense of excitement that our long journey was ending, and we would soon be seeing our families again after seven long years.

Long into the flight, the 'No Smoking' and 'Fasten Seatbelts' signs lit up, followed by an announcement from the Captain.

"This is the Captain speaking. We are to land in a little town called Meekatharra to refuel, as there is a re-fueler's strike in Perth and we need more fuel to fly on to Adelaide, our next stop after Perth. We regret this inconvenience, but it is out of our control, so sit back and relax and we will be on our way as soon as possible."

11

Australia, Home Again

We duly landed at Meekatharra, a little town in the outback with a population of about 200 people. It is rumoured that although the landing was smooth, the weight of the 747 crumpled the runway, but I cannot verify this. We sat in stifling heat as there was no air conditioning due to the engines being shut down to refuel and even smoking was not allowed, much to the chagrin of the smokers on board. These were the days when smoking was permitted on aeroplanes.

We watched through our window as a man some 30 feet below us pumped fuel into the tanks using a rotary hand pump. His arms must have looked like Popeye's by the time he had pumped eight drums of fuel to allow us to become airborne again. This operation had taken some two hours, and finally the Captain restarted the engines and we roared down the runway into the dawn of another hot summer day in Australia. Shortly thereafter, the seatbelt sign came on and we landed at the world's most remote capital city, Perth.

We were met by several relatives who had been waiting in the airport for hours due to our unplanned detour to Meekatharra. After exchanging greetings, we said we were tired and departed for a long sleep at our hotel, which had been arranged by Ray's new employer.

It was only later that morning, Christmas Day of 1974, when we learned that the town of Darwin in the far north of the country had been virtually demolished by Cyclone Tracy with 71 fatalities. Darwin had a population of 48,000 people at that time, 10,000 of whom had fled by car to escape the approaching storm. In the aftermath, with all utilities out of commission and little food and shelter available, a massive airlift was organised to evacuate the town's residents. In the five ensuing days, 25,000 people were flown out of Darwin, culminating in 674 people packed in one 747 jet being flown to safety. This was a record at that time, achieved by stripping all the seats from the giant aircraft and seating the dishevelled passengers directly on the floor.

The next few days passed in a flurry of visits with relatives and friends we hadn't seen in over seven years. The children had all grown much taller, and most adults had grown portlier. They were all charmed by Stephen's outgoing personality, humour and American accent. Once again, we were a novelty. Our own accent had changed only mildly; however, we used words that were not in common usage in Australia at that time, and everyone would laugh at everything we said, like 'automobile' in place of car or 'ketchup' in place of tomato sauce.

The frenzy gradually died down and we settled into the business of adjusting to shops closing at noon on Saturdays, and the Post Office not opening at all until Monday. We had become used to being able to shop around the clock, with department stores open every day till 9:00 PM in the USA. The possibility of Sunday trading in Perth was still 30 years in the future, although Saturday trading would be extended to 5:00 PM in a few years' time.

Meanwhile, Ray had been transferred to run a gold mine on the other side of the country. Stephen and I stayed with Ray's mother, the

Glasses Nana. Although she was very welcoming to us both, living there was not easy for Stephen as her house was not wheelchair friendly. It was difficult to manoeuvre him in his hired wheelchair through the narrow doorways and small bathroom.

After many enquiries, we were approached by social workers with the view to placing Stephen in a facility caring for handicapped children, and soon he entered a lovely large converted house with ocean views at Mosman Park, a popular beachside suburb. Here Stephen made new friends – Debbie, who was also burdened with brittle bones, and Monica, who was born a Thalidomide baby without arms and legs. They would congregate in the music room where Stephen would play Beatles music until after midnight. A few other children enjoyed classical compositions, which Stephen also knew well and played in quiet moments of reflection.

There were constant requests from everyone wanting Stephen to record Beatles music onto tapes for them with his recording equipment. He loved doing this and taught himself many useful music studio techniques. It would take him hours of work to get the sound perfect. He would not accept anything less than perfect for the finished product. I would bring more tapes for him to record on each time I visited him. With his school studies and music recording, Stephen stayed busy, which helped keep his mind active and his pain tolerable.

It was very comforting to meet the friendly and welcoming staff caring for Stephen. Knowing that Stephen was being cared for and in good hands was a great relief, while Ray was away working on a mine in New South Wales on the east coast of Australia. Stephen was once again immensely popular with the staff and patients at his new home. At shower time, Stephen and the young orderlies would sing at the top of their lungs. It was the highlight of his day. He met an orderly named Geoff and his wife Fran, who became his lifelong friends and often took Stephen to church or invited him to stay in their home.

Stephen kept everyone enthralled with his tales of travel and experiences in America. He had seen firsthand such things that were only available at that time in the USA. A teacher was assigned for him to continue his studies in math, English and German. I visited Stephen every day to make sure he was doing well. Because I had studied German for three years at college in America, I was able to help him with the language and assist him in his homework. We had so much fun when he mimicked the German accent.

Ray's work on the goldmine was difficult, as it was the first gold mine of its type in Australia. Shortly before we left America, Ray had been sent to the famous Homestake Mine in Lead, South Dakota, to learn about the revolutionary Carbon-in-Pulp method for recovering gold from cyanide solutions. He spent three days at what was the largest and deepest gold mine in North America at the time, learning about the process. The Australian mine, however, was poorly designed and needed constant repairs and modifications to keep it running. Ray would work long into the nights and then drive thirty miles through kangaroo-infested country to his temporary home in a motel in Cobar, New South Wales.

A fully grown kangaroo can be up to 2.4 metres tall, weigh 90 kg and can hop extremely fast. They can jump up to 10 metres with every bounce. There was always the threat that they may jump onto the road and cause a serious accident. This was not an uncommon phenomenon in rural Australia. They would jump on to the road from out of bushes and become startled by the headlights of an oncoming car and freeze. An unsuspecting driver would be forced to slam their brakes or swerve into dangerous gravel, which could end disastrously for the driver. Ray was lucky that he never encountered a 'kanga' on these trips.

While he was away, Ray spent many lonely nights writing many letters to Stephen. I have chosen to replicate below one of the letters that Stephen wrote to his dad and that Ray answered on 14 March, 1975. Ray's letter echoes his love for his son.

MON

Dear Dad,

I am staying in bed today because my back hurts when I sit up. Mum rubs my back and puts a hot water bottle on it.

I will be having a test at the school so they will know what kind of books to give me. I have 3 math books to do, Algebra, Geometry and Arithmatic. I'll end up doing Arithmatic no mater what kind of Math I do. No one gets hired for drawing triangles either.

I go in the pool without my braces because I need them more when I get out than I do when I'm in the pool. I can float on my back and swim the length of the pool about 5 times.

My good leg is getting stonger so I stand on it a few minutes at a time. My hips are straitening too. My shoulders are stronger too.

When I was in the pool Friday my bad leg touched the side of the pool while I was floating and it started to staighten at my knee and that makes my rod lengthen so I tried to keep it bent and my thigh muscle came of the surface of the bone. Its getting better though.

Saturday Mum and I went to John and Helen's place. We went and had hamburgers. John said as we passed the houses on the south side of Canning bridge that thier lots cost $35,000 for being on the water. There was a road between their houses and the water. We got lost going to the drivein but we got there on time. We saw Papilon. It was about prisoners in some jungle. Dustin Hoffman made lots of money selling eyeglasses and he swallowed his money so nobody could get it. He wears glasses and limps and has that strange voice.

Steve Mcqueen mouthed off to a guard and was jailed. Hoffman sent him a coconut in prison to keep Mcqueen from starving. The guard found out that he got food so since Mcqueen didn't tell who sent it he was starved until he ate cocroaches and kept in the dark for 6 months. When he got out he visited a doctor who sold a boat to him so they could escape. Mcqueen and his friend decided to escape and Hoffman did at the last minute. They had to climb a 20 ft wall, and Hoffman broke his ankle when he landed on the other side. They ran to the boat and Hoffman says quite calmly "I got something to tell you, I broke my ankle." Then Mcqueen gets mad at him for breaking it and then they try the boat and they put their foot through it. A native builds a boat for them and they sail on a raft through 20 ft high waves...

They had to amputate Hoffmans
leg. Then they get to an Island
and Mcqueen gave a begging nun
some pearls, she lets him
stay at her house and got
the police. He stayed in jail
for 5 more years. He then got
out and was sent to Devils
Island with Hoffman. Mcqueen's
were chopped of and
Hoffman's leg was artificial.
They both jumped. Hoffman stayed
on the Island because he had
pet pigs and a garden. Mcqueen
jumped of the cliff with a
raft and made it home.
I had a good time with
John and Helen. We all laughed alot.
Sunday we went to aunty
Peggys for 2 hours.
We might go to the drive-in
next Saturday if my back is
better.
Bye for now
Love
Steve XX 80

The letter Stephen wrote to his dad

Dear Stevie. Friday 14.

Received your letter today, Friday.
Well, your letter had a lot of good news in it.
I am happy that you can go in the pool now without your braces, your legs must be much stronger. This shows definite signs of progress – start off slowly with the braces so that your muscles build up to say 33⅓% of efficiency, then go without braces to get up to 100% efficiency. Without your braces you will be able to float and swim much better but I was surprised, pleased and proud that you can swim the length of the pool 5 times. I never would have thought you would do so well so quickly. I am really proud of my boy. Of course, all that swimming is probably why your back is so sore, this means that your back muscles are building up their efficiency too. All we have to do now is swim strongly with the left arm and build up your arm and shoulder muscles and it will be all over. If you get in the middle of the pool, floating on your back and stroke with your left arm you will turn in circles and this way you will be exercising your left arm and be getting giddy at the same time. Swimming under water will be a good thing for arms, legs and lungs. In three months or so, we may be able to take the splint off your arm for good. Once the muscles build up, the bone will grow and strengthen. then goodbye Left Arm Splint! You said you can stand on your good leg for a few minutes – is this in the water or out?

Happy about your math, too. As you say, not many people get hired to draw triangles, but the mathmatics of triangles is involved in almost everything you may do in later life.

Try not to crash into the side of the pool and tear your muscles off the bone – dim dum!

I know that is very painful. I once had some muscles torn from my ribs and it hurt like hell for 3 weeks. I went to the movies the other night and saw "The Sting" again. It is a good show but there were 3,773,433 screaming kids in the theatre (or was it 3,773,434? - I can't remember now) and it was very hard to hear the movie. Glad you liked Papillon (that is the French word for butterfly) (How is your German coming on?) Do you remember the ads for Papillon on our Colour T.V in the states?

Canbelego now has 17 people living here, once there were 10,000 & 8 hotels etc. On Sunday we went to a dam near here and caught some freshwater "yabbies" or as we call them in West Aust - marron. They were big too - a lot of them about 10" long. That night we cooked them and barbecued some steak, and I drank a little of my special "medicine" and we had a good time. The men I work & mix with come from Port Augusta in S.A and we have a lot of fun together. I will take some photos of the house soon and send them to you so you can see "the Ranch." I think I will be home for Easter so we will all be together again for a few days. By that time you will propably be runnin & jumpin etc. It is really hot here today and luckily there is no breeze, otherwise there would be tons of dust blowing around. You have to drive with all the windows up & the vents closed and you sweat like crazy. Air filters on my Holden Kingswood Station Sedan (latest model) have to be changed once a week or the engine gets no air to burn the petrol and the engine wont run. Well Stevie boy, will close now you should get this about next thursday, so until I see you at Easter, keep up the good work and remember I love you & am proud of you

all my love, Dad xxxoooxx

The letter Ray wrote to Stephen

With Stephen settled in his new care facility, I decided to go back to University to continue studying for a degree in psychology. I sent for my transcript from the University of Alabama in Huntsville and presented it to the Western Australia Institute of Technology (now named Curtin University). After viewing my transcript, the

Administrator indicated that the subjects I had taken in America served as prerequisites and in order to continue my studies I would need to start the semester with statistics as a subject. I found this course difficult but interesting.

Eventually I had to give up my plans seeking a degree in psychology. Stephen was going through a series of stress fractures to his arms or legs or both. My mother was showing early signs of dementia and was now living in a nursing home. Between trying to study, managing medical appointments for Stephen and visiting my mother, I was constantly on the go and often found it overwhelming. Although I was disappointed at abandoning my studies, I felt enormous relief too, for this enabled me to focus on my priorities, which were Stephen and my mother.

I had bought a small car to drive directly to my destinations rather than rely on public transport, which never seemed to go where I wanted to go. This was instrumental in paying visits to my mother and her sister, my Aunt Peg. Most of my cousins were married and had children, and Aunt Peg's main role was chief babysitter, a pastime she cherished.

From November 1975 to January 1976, Stephen was in and out of hospital. His condition deteriorated with fractures to his arms and legs. The worst bit was when he had to go in for surgery on his left leg while having his right arm in a cast and his left arm in a permanent brace. I felt dejected by the turn of events, thinking life was always one step forward and two steps back. Ray and I hurried to his side the moment he awoke from the surgery to his left leg. His face had the usual white-as-a-sheet post-operative pallor. With blurry eyes and the aftereffects of anaesthetic, Stephen shakily lifted his head and looked down at his foot.

"They've put my foot on wrong," he mumbled in a drowsy voice.

I quickly told him that it only looked that way because of the bulky bandages, but I cannot remember speaking with the doctor about this. The results of operations were not always predictable due to the fact that Stephen's bones were malleable due to OI. Post-surgery, his foot was turned to the right towards the other leg. Once again, my heart broke into pieces at his sad state. I was filled with despair. Ray helped us focus on the positive, speaking about how Stephen must get strong again to go swimming and that there were more adventures and sights yet to see.

In November 1975, while Stephen was in hospital for surgery, Beatle Paul McCartney came to Perth to perform in a concert.

Stephen was tied up in bed in traction and too sick to go to the concert. I wrote a letter to the concert organisers, the Perth Entertainment Centre, asking them if it would be possible for Paul McCartney to visit Stephen in hospital as that would boost his morale. I explained that Stephen was a big fan of the Beatles and Paul was his favourite artist, adding that Stephen had every book and recording of the Beatles and Paul McCartney. I was trying to make it impossible for them to say 'no'. We did not say anything to Stephen, however, in case my request came to nothing.

Lo and behold! While we were visiting Stephen the next day, who should turn up beside his bed? None other than Paul McCartney's manager, who handed Stephen a folder with signed autographs and best wishes from Paul and Linda and the band members.

This was a highlight of Stephen's young life and a memory he treasured for years.

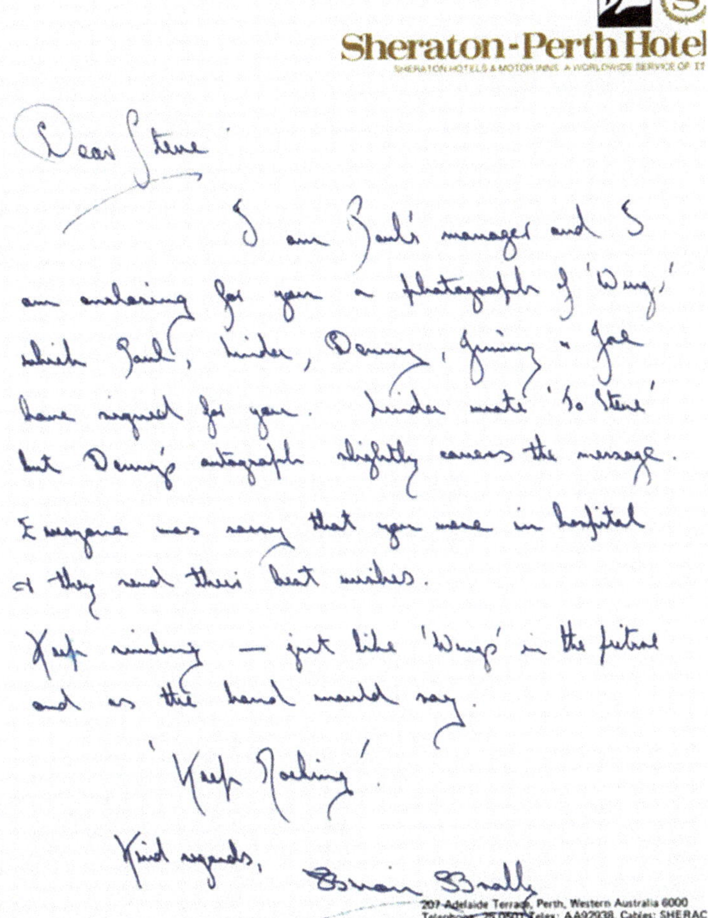

Sheraton-Perth Hotel
SHERATON HOTELS & MOTOR INNS, A WORLDWIDE SERVICE OF IT

Dear Steve

I am Paul's manager and I am enclosing for you a photograph of 'Wings,' which Paul, Linda, Denny, Jimmy & Joe have signed for you. Linda wrote 'To Steve' but Denny's autograph slightly covers the message.

Everyone was sorry that you were in hospital & they send their best wishes.

Keep smiling — just like 'Wings' in the picture and as the band would say

'Keep Rocking'.

Kind regards,

Brian Brolly

207 Adelaide Terrace, Perth, Western Australia 6000
Telephone: 25 0501 Telex: AA92938, Cables: SHERAC

One day when I was sitting in a chair beside Stephen's bed in hospital, there was a young boy in a bed behind me who was also in traction. This little boy was being very boisterous. I looked at Stephen and saw an alarmed look on his face and my instinct was to spin around quickly. The little boy was on the edge of his bed about to fall off. I quickly put both arms under him and placed him gently back on to his bed.

“That was lucky, Mum,” Stephen said.

I thought about how quickly I had acted in other times in Port Hedland when he had broken his upper arm and again in Wyoming when he had fractured his forearm and I had held his arm together until we arrived at the hospital. It seemed that I had developed a sixth sense and intuitively knew what to do in a variety of emergency situations. These episodes left me feeling sick for days, with flashbacks of panic-stricken moments.

Stephen was in hospital for months. All the nurses fell in love with him. They made a fuss over him and attended to his every need. They would play games around his bed, having so much fun. They played an instrumental role in his recovery by making him laugh, and he in turn made them laugh with his quick wit. His mimicking of American accents and narrating stories of his many adventures had them all in stitches of laughter.

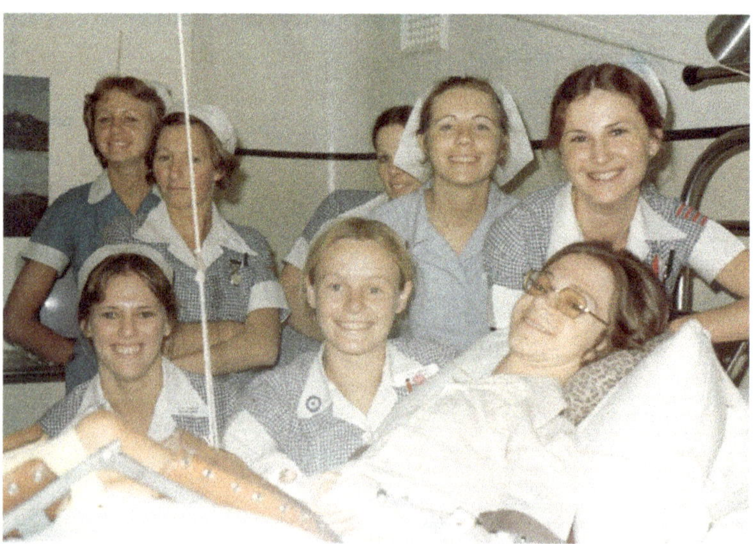

Stephen in hospital with the nurses

When Stephen came home from the hospital, we got him an electric wheelchair to get around in. An extension was attached to the chair to keep his right leg straight and supported. He was able to get around by himself. He would go at breakneck speed to wherever he wanted to go. Once again, I was filled with dread that something would happen to him, but he knew what he was doing, so I kept my fear to myself. He even went to high school for a while with other young teenagers, which did him a world of good and allowed him to experience a bit of normal school life once more.

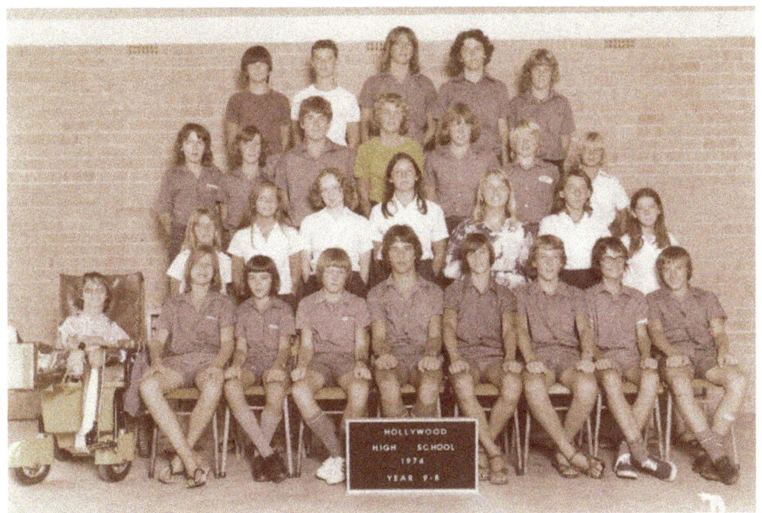

Stephen and his class of 1976

After two years in Australia, we became restless and wanted to go back to America. We could not adjust to the different lifestyle. Most annoying was the shops closing at midday. People who worked all week from 9 to 5 would try to do grocery shopping, buy furniture or home appliances, fix car problems or even fill the car up with petrol within just the four hours on Saturday mornings, as everything was closed on Sundays.

I was bewildered and frustrated that the public did not know any different and just accepted things for how they were. I would try to inform them how life was so convenient in America. At my work, they would refer to me as, "here comes in America!" Even though everyone loved the stories of our adventures and begged for more, they saw me as complaining and told me to 'get back to America then'. Therefore, with mixed feelings we decided to travel back to America. Today, the lifestyle in Australia is somewhat similar to that in America, but it took 30 long years to catch up.

Stephen's Australian-made electric wheelchair would not be suitable for use in America. We had an idea for a carrier design that could better support Stephen's legs. He could not bend his right knee yet since his surgery. Ric Renton, a very clever mechanically minded man who worked at fixing broken wheelchairs in the care facility's workshop, went home and quickly made the carrier we had described in his dad's shed. Support cushions were put in for his back and along the full length of the carrier for his legs. We could put Stephen in his carrier on the back seat of any car to transport him around. By this

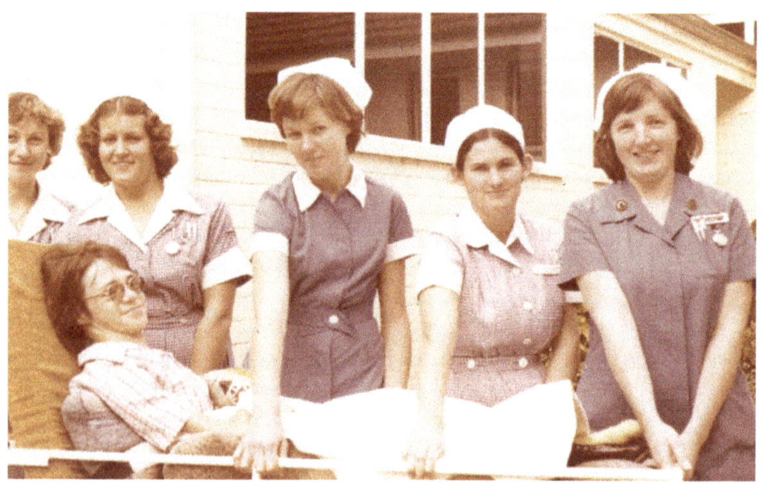

August 1976, Stevie back in hospital in his carrier.

time Stephen's right arm and leg were out of plasters, but he was back in hospital for a short stay to get a brace made for his right leg. He now had braces on both legs.

The following month, in September 1976, we were at Perth Airport once again saying goodbye to all our family and Stephen's good friends from his nursing home in anticipation of flying towards new unknown adventures.

PART 4: TRAVELS

STEPHEN AGE 17—20

12

Going Back to America

We flew to Sydney and on to San Francisco, where at an immigration desk an officer checked our passports and Green Cards and said, "Welcome Home."

It immediately made us less apprehensive, and we taxied to a motel near Fisherman's Wharf. This time we had no job to go to, no house, no car nor any of life's comforts, and only a small amount of money. We unpacked our three suitcases and Ray settled down with the local newspapers in search of a job. Looking for mining jobs proved fruitless.

Meanwhile, I was feeling disoriented. Here I was once again, thousands of miles from home and facing the unknown. I was tired of the rigmarole of our life being repeated in an endless cycle of wondering what would come next. Inevitably, in the future, there was more to come. The fun of the new adventure temporarily lost its gloss, but I tried to stay positive. I turned the television on for Stephen and much to his delight, he discovered an episode of The Monkees that showcased the four lads in 'Beatlesesque' mode with songs that had similar harmonies, chord progressions and musical style to that of Beatles music. Thereafter, he never missed an episode. They became one of his favourite music groups.

After three weeks without prospects, Ray and I thought to call our friends Upendra and Maria Roy, who now lived in Oak Ridge, Tennessee – the Atomic City, so named as this was where work on the Atom bomb was conducted in World War II. At that time, entry and exit was strictly controlled. The township was nestled in a valley between two large hills, in case of an atomic explosion.

On hearing of our return to America and our plight, Maria insisted we come to Oak Ridge to stay with them until we found work. This was good news to us, despite the fact that Oak Ridge was some 2,465 miles or 3,967 kilometres east of our present location.

Ray set out to purchase a car and eventually found a $1,200 Studebaker Station Wagon that could easily transport us, our three suitcases and Stephen in his carrier to the other side of the country. Stephen could not bend his knees anymore and his legs were locked in braces straight out in front of him. Ray would carry one end of the frame and I would carry the other to wherever we wanted to go. This was difficult, but at least we could take him everywhere with us.

The next morning, we settled our three-week motel bill and proceeded on our journey. The wagon went well and we made good progress, averaging 600 miles per day. We stayed overnight in Dollar Inns, as they were cheap, comfortable and clean. We dined royally on a mix of McDonalds (Stephen's beloved 'Golden Arches'), Arby's, Kentucky Fried Chicken, and at breakfast places such as Denny's and IHOP (International House of Pancakes).

At one petrol stop, Ray and I headed for the rest rooms at the same time, leaving Stephen in the car to safeguard our belongings. This was in the days when an attendant fuelled the car, checked the oil and cleaned the windscreen. When Ray returned, the attendant pointed to some oil on the ground and said that the shock absorbers were damaged and could cause irreparable damage if they were not fixed.

He pointed out that he was a good 'Christian' man and wouldn't take advantage of a young family, so a little while later, with new shock absorbers and $150 dollars lighter, we went on our way. To this day, however, we are not convinced that the repairs were necessary.

The trip was exciting and we enjoyed the drive on Interstate 40 East, passing through Arizona, New Mexico, Texas, Oklahoma, Arkansas and on to Nashville in Tennessee.

While we were driving along the freeway in Oklahoma, I saw a sign reading 'Visit Cowboy Hall of Fame' with directions to the museum. We made a slight detour to the museum and what we saw there made a lasting impression on our minds. We were able to hire a suitable wheelchair with leg extensions to push Stephen around the museum.

In the atrium of the museum, there was a large beautiful white sculpture of a Native American Indian looking sadly defeated on his weary horse poised at the edge of a precipice. His hair and the horse's tail were blowing forward, the horse standing with one hoof off the ground as if about to take a step. The statue was called End of the Trail. It has become one of the most familiar sculptures of the American West, depicting an Indian who has come to the end of the trail, symbolizing the end of the Indians' world as they knew it since the white man took all their land away.

The sculpture was originally developed by James Earle Fraser in 1894. He won the Wanamaker Prize at the Paris American Artists' Association in 1898. Fraser developed the statue based on the extensive interactions he'd had with Native Americans during his childhood. He came to believe that the Indians had been treated unfairly by white men. In his memoirs, Fraser wrote:

As a boy, I remembered an old Dakota trapper saying, "The Indians will someday be pushed into the Pacific Ocean." Later the idea occurred to me of making an Indian who represented his race "reaching the end of the trail, at the edge of the Pacific."

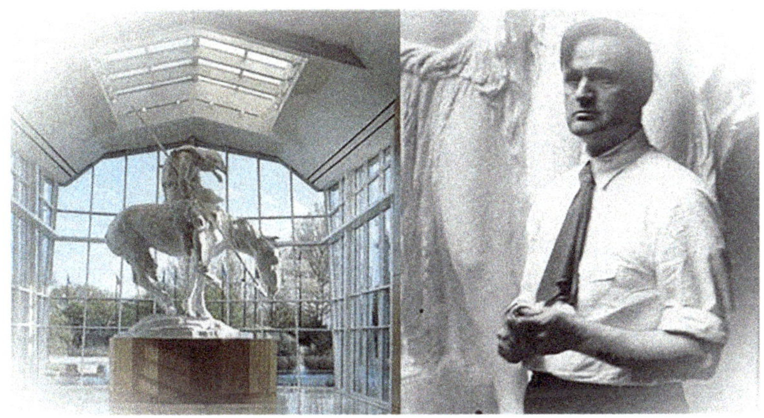

The End of the Trail Sculpture stands 18 feet tall & James Earle Fraser, the Sculptor

History tells that the summer of 1877 brought tragedy to the Nez Perce Indian tribe. By October, winter was approaching. There was a lack of food and supplies and the effects of travelling over 1500 miles over rough territory began to take its toll. Some of the tribe had been removed to a reservation. The remaining Nez Perce protested. Nez Perce leaders decided to look for a new home along the way towards Canada. Many battles took place with the Army. At the last battle at Bear Paw Mountain, Montana Territory, Chief Joseph surrendered his remaining forces. In his surrender speech, Chief Joseph concluded saying to his Chiefs.

"I am tired. My heart is sick and sad from where the sun now stands; I will fight no more forever."

Since learning about Indians in Wyoming, Stephen found the museum and Indian stories very interesting, especially he was in awe of the huge white Sculpture.

We finally arrived at Oak Ridge on the fourth day.

We were greeted warmly by our good friends. We were surprised to learn that Upendra's contract with the Atomic Energy Commission had ended. This meant two families without income were sharing a two-bedroom apartment. We were all comfortable with each other and took this time to share our respective adventures since we had parted company in Huntsville, Alabama, four years ago.

At this time, the multimillionaire Hunt brothers were actively buying silver in an effort to control the market. Upendra and Ray discussed spending $1,000 each to buy Silver Futures but desisted in the interests of saving money. Had they followed their gut and bought and sold before the inevitable crash, they would have been multimillionaires also over the years. Alas, it was not to be.

Stephen was 16 years old and delighted in talking about all things technical. Ray and Upendra joined in discussing everything under the sun with him. Stephen was especially enthralled with Upendra's stories of when he worked at Oak Ridge, because the atomic centre was of great interest to him. Maria was well-versed in current politics, and Stephen would mimic her German accent and Upendra's Indian accent. We would all be in fits of laughter. Upendra, with his brilliant mind, would pace up and down reciting mathematical formulas. To Stephen's amusement, on one occasion the globe burned out on the coffee table lamp. Upendra bent down to turn the lamp switch on and exclaimed, "Oh, the lamp is broken," thinking the lamp had to be replaced and not the light bulb. He continued pacing and muttering "x plus y equals…" Stephen couldn't help giggling. It was like witnessing a circus unfolding: with two unemployed mad scientists, Maria's political observations and Stephen's witty commentary, all taking their turns at centre stage.

During this time, Ray noticed an advertisement in the local newspaper for a welding inspector at the Atomic Energy Commission Plant in Oak Ridge. He applied and secured an interview with the Chief Engineer. When he returned, he told us he was given a facility tour after a small conversation. He was in awe of the pulsing blue lights of the atomic core in the main building. However, Ray had been offered a salary he deemed inadequate, so he had thanked the Engineer for the tour and returned to the apartment still unemployed.

About three weeks into our enforced stay in Oak Ridge, the local paper advertised for a metallurgist to run a gold mine in Nevada. Ray rang the advertiser and was hired over the phone. He accepted reluctantly as Tonopah, Nevada, was some 2,161 miles back the way we had recently travelled. We packed our belongings into the station wagon again and carried Stephen into the car. I tearfully said goodbye to our generous hosts, and we turned westward on Interstate 40 towards another new adventure.

We were on the road about an hour from Oak Ridge when we saw a car in front of us suddenly make a sharp turn, catapulting over the guard rail, landing right side up and bursting into flames. We came to a sudden halt as did the cars behind us. We all looked on helplessly as an arm slowly rose up behind the front passenger window, all blackened against a background of yellow fire. The scene has stayed forever lodged in my memory. We eventually got back into our car crying and with a heavy heart continued very carefully on our journey.

Arriving in Kansas, we were lost. We drove around till we saw a little girl about 10 years old walking on the footpath. Ray pulled over and asked her, “Where are we?”

She bellowed loudly in her southern accent. "You're in Salaaana Kaynsis, misterrrrr."

Translation: "You're in Salina, Kansas, mister."

I still hear this little girl in my mind, and it remains a fond memory. Stephen would mimic her so well and make us and everyone laugh.

A few days later, we arrived in Tonopah, Nevada, and met the company representative at the Mizpah Hotel. He escorted us to our new home, a 40 by 12 feet (12.192 x 3.6576 metres) long trailer home! But it proved quite comfortable.

Ray started work the next day and met four other employees on a previous mine site that had prospered in the 1800s. The equipment that remained was rusted and not at all suited to the requirements of gold processing. Ray indicated his concerns but was told to do his best and get it running for six months as taxation credits were being claimed. Ray and his crew worked 10–15 hours per day overcoming seemingly insurmountable odds to keep the plant running. Winter had set in by then and the flat prairie land was exposed to every icy breeze that came along.

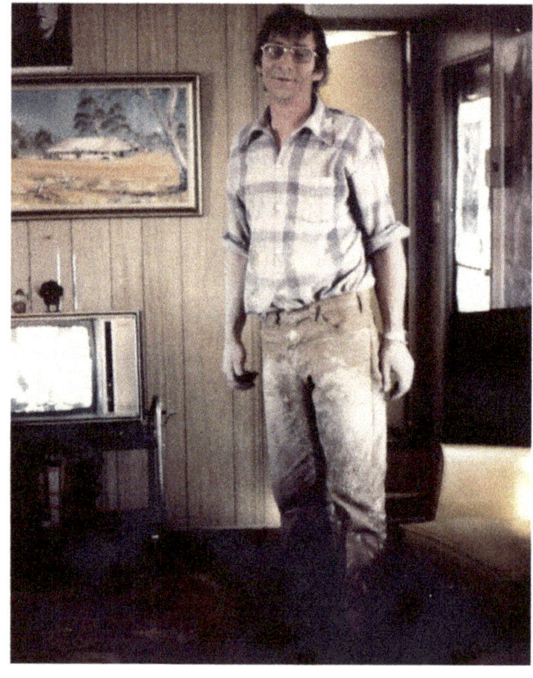

Ray home from the mine in our trailer home

We were truly now in the hub of stories about the American Wild West. I could not get enough of the historical events and people that had lived here long ago. No doubt I had inherited a passion for cowboys, horses and this turbulent era from my father. He would have been an impressionable young man in the early 1900s. During those years, there was a worldwide interest in the history and stories of gunfighters, gamblers and the American West. This was fuelled by the plethora of Western movies at that time.

The Mizpah Hotel is a member of Historic Hotels of America. It was named after the Mizpah Mine which in 1900 was the largest producer of silver and gold in the area. The name Mizpah is Hebrew for "watchtower" and signifies a promise that two Old Testament biblical figures made when they built a tower that separated the borders of their territories. They promised to never cross those borders to do evil to each other and the tower was built to reach God, who was the witness to their agreement.

The hotel construction began in 1905. It features the "Wyatt Earp bar," named after Wyatt Earp (1848 – 1929). He and his brother Virgil were known foremost for the famous gunfight at the O.K. Corral in Tombstone, Arizona in 1881.

Wyatt moved from town to town across the West, earning his living as a saloonkeeper, gunslinger, gambler, miner, and frontier lawman. He moved to Tonopah in 1902. Although Wyatt left Tonopah before the Mizpah hotel was completed, a bar was named after him. He later served as a Deputy U.S. Marshal in Nevada. After his death, aged 80, the newspaper "The Tombstone Epitaph," reported that Tom Mix, a close friend of Wyatt cried during the funeral service. Tom Mix was a silent movie star (and my father's hero).

We were unaware then that soon we would be visiting this historical town of Tombstone in Arizona.

Goldfield, now a ghost town was made famous by Wyatt and Virgil Earp. Virgil Earp and his wife Allie went to Goldfield, a new gold-mining boom town in 1904, a half hour drive from Tonopah, where brother Wyatt was running a saloon, and had previously served briefly as a U.S. Deputy Marshal. Virgil led an adventurous life as a Civil War Veteran and he participated in the gunfight at the O.K. Corral in Tombstone, Arizona. A few months after the gunfight, Virgil was shot in his back and left arm by friends of slain outlaws. He was permanently maimed. His assailants were let off for lack of evidence. After this, he carried a "break-top" revolver which could be reloaded with one hand. These experiences would have been fuel for great stories among the miners.

Virgil later became U.S Marshal for Esmeralda County in Nevada; shortly after he was slowed down by pneumonia. It was difficult to enforce the law from his bed, and after 6 months of illness Virgil died on October 19, 1905, aged 62. Virgil was known as one of the most daring and adventurous of Western pioneers. He was a good-hearted man who helped to build the West.

Jack Dempsey – 1895 – 1983 was one of the world's greatest boxing legends. Some of his earliest matches were in Tonopah and Goldfield. He was inducted into the International Boxing Hall of Fame in1954. There is a room named after him in the Mizpah Hotel. He died in New York City, of heart failure aged 87.

Howard Robard Hughes Jr. 1905 – 1976 was an American entrepreneur, known during his life as one of the most financially successful individuals in the world. Prompted by his obsession for privacy, he married actress Jean Peters in a secret ceremony in the remote mining town of Tonopah, Nevada. She was 30 and Hughes was 51. Later in life, he became known for his eccentric behavior and reclusive lifestyle which was caused in part by a worsening obsessive–compulsive disorder and chronic pain from a plane crash. He died of kidney failure on an emergency flight from Acapulco to Houston, Texas in 1976, aged 70.

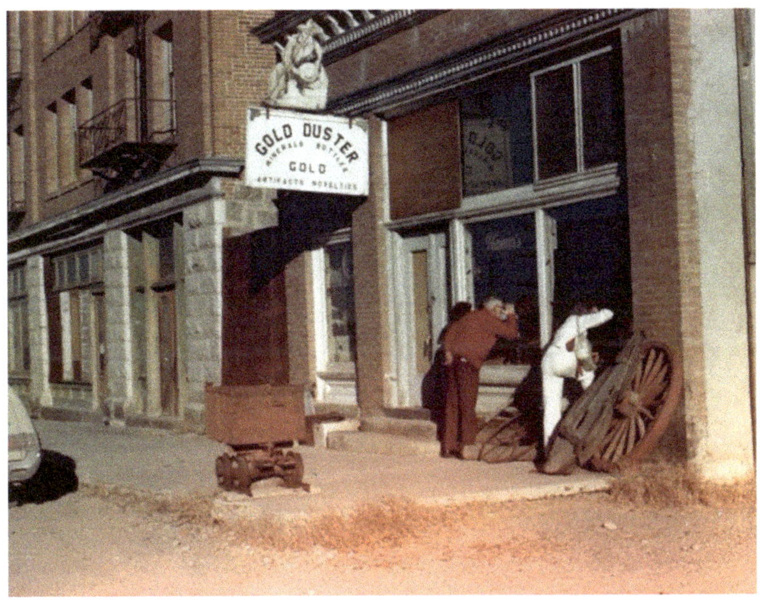

Looking into the Goldfield Hotel window

13

Happy Trails

Stephen, then 17 years of age, was being home tutored by a high school teacher who was amazed at his learning capabilities, general knowledge, and humorous outlook on life. She convinced Stephen to take a test to determine his I.Q. Imagine our surprise when later she knocked on the door greeting us with excitement, proclaiming "Do you know your son is a genius? He has an I.Q. of 180!"

I didn't know what that meant, so she then drew the bell curve and explained that his score was in the uppermost end of the curve. His score was amongst the masterminds of the world! Albert Einstein was 160. I was elated thinking that my boy's brain would serve to get him through life despite his bone condition.

Also, at this time a preacher came to our trailer door and after a long chat about God, Stephen concluded that he was saved. His faith had been reinforced by the preacher. I was sceptical because his visit seemed aimed at selling bibles. However, it was Stephen's choice and I thought he was old enough to hold on to his own personal beliefs of faith.

As time went by, the mine settled down a little and the cyanide dam was commissioned. Warning signs reading 'Cyanide: Keep Away' were put up everywhere as efforts were continuously made to produce some gold. One morning, Ray arrived at work to find 12 dead cows near the cyanide pond. He inspected the ear tags required on all 'open range' cattle and telephoned the ranch indicated on the tag. The owner was not too pleased on hearing the fate of his 12 steers and drove with his two noticeably big sons to the mine. He collected the ear tags from the dead steers. Ray arranged for the earth mover to dig a large hole and bury the dead cattle. The ranchers built a reed fence around the pond and returned home.

Two weeks later, the same thing happened, only this time 18 cattle were involved. The rancher was furious now, and the ear tags were again collected and the corpses buried. An air of great tension evolved over these occurrences, but the rancher conceded that the fence his sons had built was no match for thirsty steers and that the reclaimed ear tags would allow him to graze new cattle on the range. Before parting, he invited Ray to come visit his ranch up in the mountains surrounding Tonopah.

The next weekend, the three of us made our way some 25 miles from Tonopah to the ranch which was home to the family, including the two hefty sons, their wives and a couple of grandsons. The eldest grandson, about seven years old, was called Buckwheat (or Bucky for short,). Buckwheat is a type of nutritious cereal grain. In later years, we would call Stephen 'Bucky' for fun as a reminder of that happy time. We were entertained by the sons' roping, throwing calves, and branding. Soon Ray was invited to take his turn. Despite him wearing 'the Australian uniform' of thongs and shorts, since it was a hot summer's day, he remained uninjured and downed his calf in a rare show of strength and bravado. Stephen and I were delighted at the goings-on as we had never been in the company of real cowboys before.

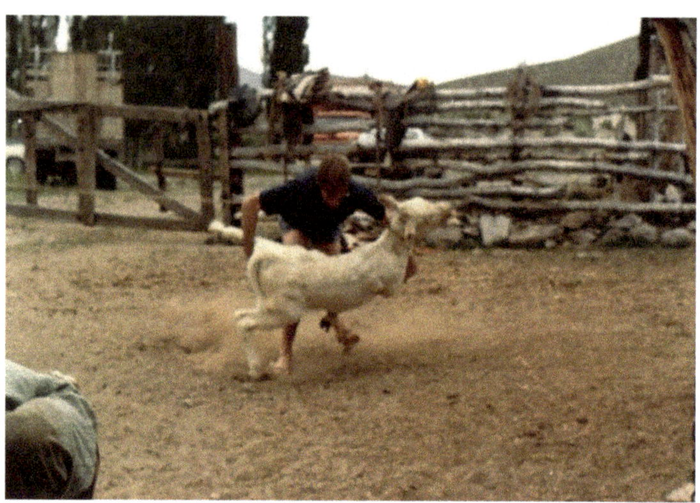

Ray learning how to prepare a calf for branding

More excitement was yet to come as Ray and I were invited to take a little ride, on what we were assured were tranquil horses. Ray suspected this was a set-up. He grabbed a handful of the horse's mane in a death grip, wrapping the reins around his other hand. The ranchers laughed to each other and we set off at a casual walk across the paddock. Suddenly, Ray's horse took off, galloping helter-skelter towards a boundary fence. Ray was leaning back as far as he could, legs stretched forward in the stirrups, hanging on for dear life. The horse headed straight for a fence and came to a slithering stop mere inches from the railings. Ray stayed on and was much relieved when the cowboys rescued him from his predicament. We all had a good laugh and proceeded to have a most enjoyable barbecue with our newfound friends.

As we were leaving, this wonderful family gave us a beautiful ginger cat as company for Stephen. We named him Oscar. He loved to play in the snow on the back porch of our trailer. When Ray and I would climb a small mountain at the back of our trailer, a frequent ritual, Oscar was eager to lead the way.

Ray's mine was on a flat area of a wide valley not far from the Air Force Base at Indian Springs in Area 51 north of Las Vegas. The base was shrouded in mystery, and it was here that many attack strategies were developed. It was a training ground for low-flying, radar-evading tactics and had some frightening aspects to its training missions.

Ray experienced this firsthand when one day, a jet fighter raced overhead, 50 feet (15.24 metres) above the ground. All that Ray knew was that he was suddenly enveloped in the sound of screaming jet engines just overhead; he later told me that he had stood totally paralysed until the noise receded. In the distance he saw the fighter plane tip its wings from side to side, as if the pilot was having a great old time. Ray saw coyotes racing across the flat scared almost to death, howling devilishly as they headed for shelter.

Our trailer would shake when the pilots broke the sound barrier, resulting in a loud bang from the jet's sonic boom. Stephen was thrilled to bits every time this happened – on a regular basis and normally at 10 AM. In time, everyone on the mine was prepared for it and would wave to the pilot for the one to two seconds he was in the area. Those pilots certainly were very brave lads to be flying that fast, so close to the ground.

The mine was an ongoing headache and was built in such a manner that it would never be operational. Long hours of work day and night, with snowstorms and biting winds, took a toll on the workforce. After six months, Ray had meetings with the owners, advising them to abandon the project which had already cost two million dollars with little prospect of a return. The mine owners agreed to close the mine, thanked the workforce for their extraordinary efforts and paid everyone a small bonus. We were free again to continue our adventures in this vast land.

The weekend before the mine closed, Ray gathered us together and drove the worn-out station wagon into Las Vegas to use as a trade-in for a new vehicle. The pistons were damaged due to driving on the mine. The fine residue from the original treatment had been sucked in through the air filter and had acted like sandpaper, grinding down the pistons. The trip into Vegas was not without incident; two stops had to be made to top up the engine oil with a total of four litres. Stephen said that he could see a fine stream of oil blowing out the exhaust that grew larger the faster we drove. Luckily for us, Stephen always had a talent for noticing things we were oblivious to.

We pulled into a service station to add a little fuel to the tank and as we stopped, a radiator hose blew out. It cost $120 to be replaced, which in the '70s was a lot of money. We then began the hunt for a roomy van-type vehicle which would accommodate Stephen in his carrier frame and allow him to see everything as we travelled. A brand-new vehicle would eliminate breakdown worries. Having shuttled back and forth from inspecting Ford, Chevrolet, and Chrysler models, we finally settled on a Chevy van and drove back to Tonopah all happy. How fortunate we were to have the foresight to buy that van only four days before the mine closure.

My brother Tom had recently arrived from Australia wanting to see America and was staying with us in Tonopah. He joined in the evening discussions as to where we should go in search of Ray's next employment. Eventually, we decided to head to Houston, Texas, as this was a booming area at that time. We thought we deserved a holiday and agreed to drive to the north west to visit Seattle in

Washington State. This would take us across several other States and closer to our aim of visiting every one of the 50 that make up the United States of America. We loaded up our shiny new van with Stephen in his carrier on the back seat, allowing him a good view of everything as we drove along.

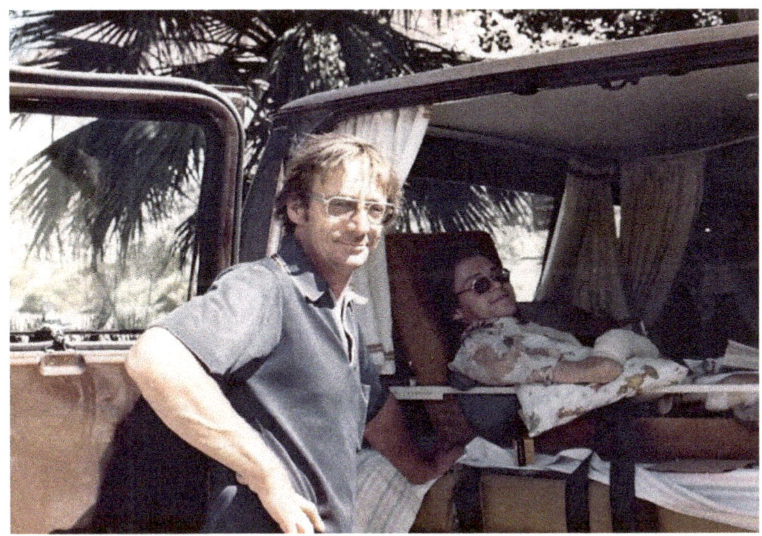

Driver and Navigator

Despite our unemployed status, we headed off on our expedition. We were in no hurry, believing that everything would turn out all right in the end. Initially, we headed to Salt Lake City, where we made a stop to revisit the Mormon Tabernacle and then went on to Yellowstone National Park in Wyoming. We left this beautiful park through the top exit into Montana, turned westward through Idaho and eventually arrived in Seattle, Washington.

We settled into a motel for the night, eagerly anticipating sightseeing around this beautiful green city. The next morning, we travelled the well-known tourist routes through the city. Then, we all rode in the elevator to the top of the Seattle Space Needle. Ray carried Stephen while I carried a small fold-up stool for Stephen to rest his legs – he still could not bend his legs. We ate lunch in the revolving restaurant and marvelled at the spectacular view of the city. After this wonderful experience, we turned southward through Portland, Oregon, and homeward to Tonopah, Nevada, completing a fantastic two-week adventure.

On one unfenced stretch of a highway, as we were going through a cutting, a deer jumped from the embankment alongside the road landing onto the roof of the van. Amazingly, we could hear its feet clattering for three or four steps on the roof before it fell onto the grassy strip beside the road. It then bounded away into the forest, looking unhurt but puzzled. Further on, another deer ran across the highway and crashed into the left-hand side of our new van, denting the panelling. This poor deer did not survive the collision.

Once back in Tonopah, all hands were kept busy packing our meagre belongings into a U-Haul trailer for our new destination: Houston, Texas. Stephen would be the map navigator, a role he took very seriously.

We started out at 8 o'clock one bright sunny morning, a little apprehensive as we did not know what fate had in store for us. We decided to go via Las Vegas out to Hoover Dam as our first bucket-list item. We joined state highway 93 east and reached Hoover Dam about an hour and a half after leaving our trailer home in Tonopah. We parked in the visitor area and marvelled at the sight of this mighty structure, named after Herbert Hoover, the thirty-first President of the United States.

It was of particular interest to us, as Hoover was a mining engineer who paid several visits to Western Australia beginning in 1897. He had encouraged his British employers to purchase a mining lease, which he developed, and where he became the Superintendent of the Sons of Gwalia (Wales) gold mine in Leonora in 1898. The mine was a prolific producer, and he introduced many labour-saving practices while there. He often stayed in the Palace Hotel in Kalgoorlie, where he fell in love with a barmaid and installed a magnificent mirror in the hotel as a parting gesture when he departed in December 1898.

He returned to the United States and married his childhood sweetheart Lou Henry on 10 February, 1899. He made several more visits to Australia in the early 1900s and with several others founded the Rio Tinto Zinc Company in Broken Hill in 1905. Rio Tinto is now one of the largest mining companies in the world. On March 4, 1929, Hoover became President and served during the Depression until March 4, 1933.

Anxious to continue our journey, we piled back into the van and headed for Kingman, Arizona, 75 miles away, where we made a left turn and drove 73 miles to the Grand Canyon. We lifted Stephen in his carrier out of the van and proceeded to the various nearby vantage points to view this spectacular landscape. We were struck by the many colours of the different layers of rock and sediment, laid bare by centuries of erosion. The scene changed with the movement of the sun's position, with lengthening shadows casting their magic on the canyon walls. We were not about to trek to the bottom of the canyon but were content instead to marvel at the workings that the Colorado River had accomplished in carving this natural wonder.

Despite the urge to stay longer, we re-entered the van and headed for a night-time stopover in Phoenix, Arizona, where we had a good night's rest, delighted with all we had accomplished on our first day of travel.

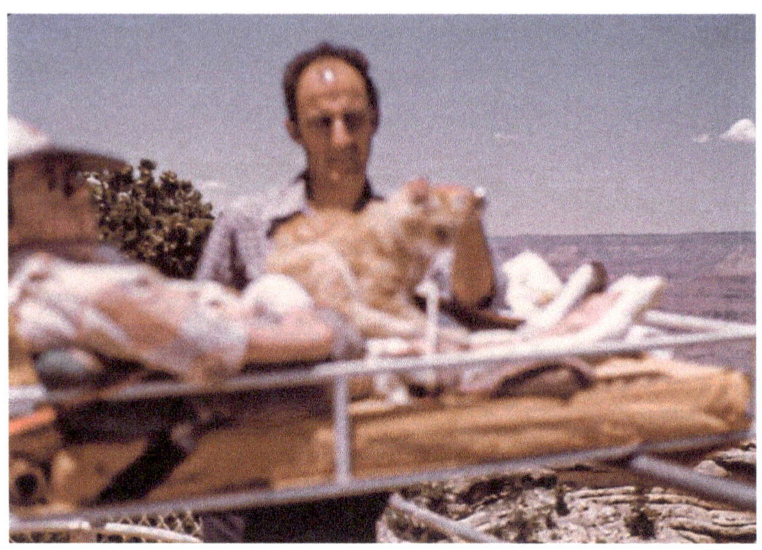

Stephen, Tom, Oscar the cat in view of the Grand Canyon

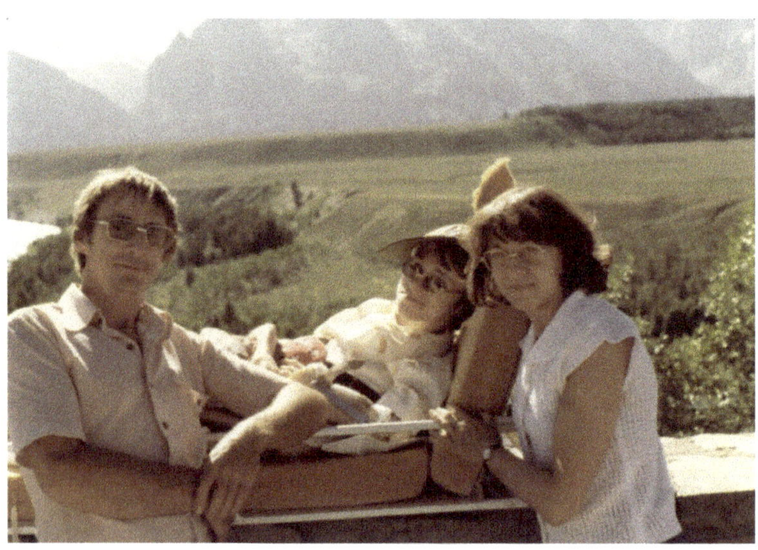

Stopping for a photo on the way to Tucson, Arizona

Next day, after a hearty breakfast at Denny's, we set off on Interstate 10 east towards our ultimate destination, Houston,

Texas. We continued on I-10 east and after two hours arrived in Tucson, Arizona, and made a unanimous decision to side-track to Tombstone, fabled in history as the site of the gunfight at the O.K. Corral. Here, on October 26, 1881, Wyatt Earp, his brothers Morgan and Virgil, along with their friend Doc Holiday, had their legendary shootout with the Clanton-McLaury gang. The fight lasted a mere 30 seconds in which time about 30 bullets were fired, resulting in the deaths of Billy Clanton, Tom and Frank McLaury and the wounding of Doc Holiday and both Morgan and Virgil Earp. Wyatt Earp was unhurt, and Ike Clanton and Billy Claiborne, the last surviving members of the outlaw gang, headed for the hills.

We carried Stephen through the famous Boot Hill Cemetery and read most of the tombstones depicting hangings, lynchings, murders and, equally notorious, the deaths of horse thieves. A majority of the occupants had died with their boots on, hence the name Boot Hill. It was a worthwhile detour as we had seen movies featuring Tombstone and the old TV series of that name, although no mention of the Earp family or the famous shootout was mentioned in the series. We bought the usual postcards and other souvenirs depicting the graveyard and took photos of the re-enactment of the shootout, staged for tourists every hour. We again loaded up and continued on the road heading for Texas.

14

Hello, Texas

After an uneventful drive to El Paso, Texas, we rested after a delicious Texas chilli supper and spent a very pleasant evening. Early the next morning, we set out for a long drive to San Antonio, Texas, home of The Alamo and the equally famous Riverwalk.

We were to stay with relatives of our rancher friends from Tonopah, Nevada, and spend a day seeing the sights of San Antonio. We had been driving for half an hour or so when a siren erupted behind us and we were told to 'pull over' by someone on a loud hailer of some type with red-and-blue flashing lights inside the van. Stephen's vantage point allowed him to keep us informed of activities to our rear, and he told us that we were to be examined by Border Patrol officials.

As El Paso is close to the Mexican border, regular patrols stop vehicles to inspect them for illegal aliens or contraband, and now it was our turn to be inspected. The patrolman was friendly as he asked for our I.D. Ray, Stephen and I produced our Green cards proving we were legally in the country.

The patrolman asked Tom to produce his ID. Since he did not have a Green card, he had to show his passport. Tom began to search through his packed bags, and after much frantic searching and placing many bags on the roadside, he finally found his passport and had it inspected. When we explained that we were going to Houston to look for work, the patrolman wished us good luck and we gathered up our belongings and again set off for our destination.

A hilarious incident took place after we arrived in San Antonio in the late afternoon, having travelled the 550 miles without further incident. We arrived at our hosts' place feeling hot and tired. Ray and my brother Tom had an argument over reversing the trailer into their driveway. Before we had even finished introducing ourselves to our hosts, Ray and Tom proceeded outside. The disagreement became more heated and the next minute, they were punching each other in senseless fury, while our hosts looked on in bewilderment. They had only a passing knowledge of English and our Spanish was non-existent; therefore, shrugs and bemused glances served as conversation.

Meanwhile, the combatants cooled down and the scuffle ended almost as soon as it had begun. Tom reversed into the driveway, unhitched the trailer and then he and Ray went off for a drink! Stephen, our hosts and I laughed about the incident, us saying how funny the looks on their faces had been while they probably wondered what kind of people we were.

Later, two children came home from school. They were bi-lingual and cross-translated for us, after which the conversation flowed freely. Stephen and I told them about us being from Australia, which they found incredulous, and we explained we had come to Houston to find work.

Ray and Tom, the two desperados, had stopped at the first cantina they saw. They had a great old time with a group of Tex-Mex barflies, singing old Spanish songs like La Poloma, Mariquita Linda, and

South of the Border in a mix of Spanglish and whatever sounded right. They came home happy but not quite drunk, displaying their bruises with pride and swearing to be mates forever.

We had a pleasant evening with our hosts who told us several statistics about the city. San Antonio's population comprised mostly Latinos. The area was made up of predominately military installations with several bases nearby, and the city had approximately 130 miles of bicycle paths. Armed with this knowledge and numerous other snippets of information, we retired to our respective beds and slept soundly, knowing that we were to be chaperoned to see the sights of San Antonio the following day.

After a substantial Mexican breakfast of 'huevos rancheros', refried beans and strong black coffee, our hostess and her two children took us on a tour of San Antonio. We first went to the old Spanish mission known worldwide as The Alamo, so named after the cottonwood trees (Alamo in Spanish) growing nearby. We felt very humble being at the site where Colonels William B Travis and James Bowie, together with Davy Crocket and others, had succumbed to the forces led by General Antonio Lopez de Santa Anna.

The Alamo had formerly been a mission named Mission de San Antonio de Valero after St Anthony de Padua, built in 1718 by Spanish Franciscan friars in order to convert the local Indians to Christianity. The construction of the mission had begun in May 1744. It was built on the banks of the San Antonio River. The mission represented a stronghold during the time that Santa Anna was claiming Texas as Mexican territory and was defended to the death by loyal 'Texans'. David Crocket was a former congressman from Tennessee and prior to that, a famous frontiersman. Jim Bowie was the inventor of the infamous Bowie Knife, a huge weapon that was too heavy for the average man to wield.

The Alamo was under siege from February 23 to March 6, 1836, and on that final day, the mission was overrun and all defendants were killed. Their bravery has been remembered in many subsequent battles by the cry 'Remember the Alamo'. We inspected the famous battle sites, including the rooms where the valiant last stand was made, and the experience had a sobering effect on us all. We decided that it was time for lunch and were taken to the beautiful Riverwalk which meanders through San Antonio.

We learned The Riverwalk was constructed beginning in 1939 as a direct result of disastrous flooding of the San Antonio River in 1921, which claimed the lives of 50 people. Several dams and flood gates were installed, leading to the decision to construct the Riverwalk, and funds were raised in 1938 to beautify the area and establish people-friendly commercial outlets. The result was a picturesque 2.5-mile long, tree-lined bustling area, replete with small bridges, restaurants, hotels and flowering gardens. The actual Riverwalk is set lower than the traffic street level, and several hotels have two entry levels, one at the street and one at the Riverwalk. Some even have the stream flowing through the lobby as these hotels were built straddling the river.

We were delighted with our surroundings and settled for the first time eating Tacos and drinking Sangria, a punch that traditionally consists of red wine and chopped fruit, and savouring other Mexican delights in this predominately Spanish heritage city. We could not resist the urge to hire a small paddle boat to explore a small stretch of the river. We loaded up Stephen in his carrier, placing him across the front of the boat, and paddled off down the river accompanied by the stares and comments of bystanders at this unusual sight. We were unfazed by this; we were accustomed to providing Stephen with opportunities to engage in normal activities, regardless of how we may appear to others.

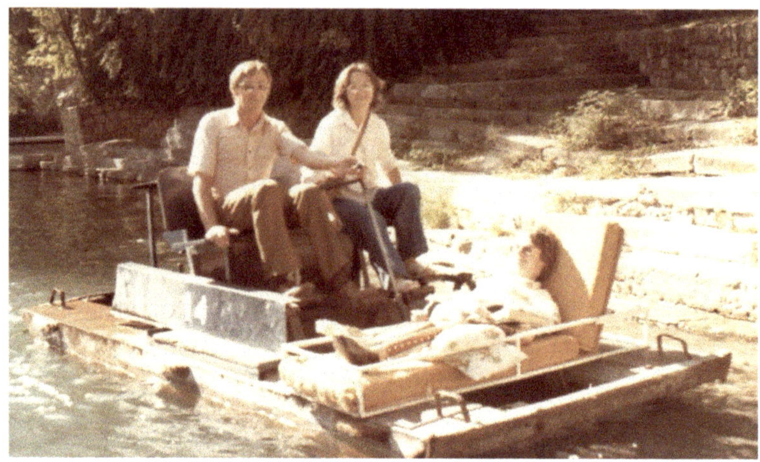

Paddling down the Riverwalk

Our cruise down the river enthralled us, as new scenery unfolded with every turn and the flower gardens were in full bloom along the riverbanks. People lined the banks, enjoying the sunny afternoon. The atmosphere felt festive, made more so by the presence of an excellent Mariachi band singing famous old Mexican songs.

Eventually, with our legs aching from steering the paddleboat, we came ashore and settled down to a meal of more tacos and tortillas with a frozen Margarita to quench the thirsts of the adults. We then loaded up our van and returned to the suburban sanctuary of our newfound friends and hosts. It was a happy little group that tumbled into bed that night, ready to continue the final leg of our journey in the morning.

Stephen was excited about finally being on the last leg of our exodus to Houston, a selection picked from a Rand McNally Road Atlas as our next place of residence. I had heard a lot about this dynamic city, and made enquiries from members of the Osteogenesis Imperfecta Chapter in Houston regarding quality of living and work potential there. I had originally selected Humble in Texas, but since it was a small community, I favoured the larger city of Houston as our next home. I had researched temporary accommodation and chosen an apartment in the South East of Houston. The occupancy was on a weekly basis, which suited our current unemployed state.

As scheduled, we bid farewell to our Mexican friends, knowing full well that we would probably never meet again, and re-joined Interstate 10 for the 190-mile run north-west to Houston. There was a growing sense of excitement, tempered with a little fear, as we approached this large city, with only a faint idea of how to find our apartment or contend with the increasing volume of traffic. Stephen's instructions served us well and the road signage made it easy to find the correct exit. After some three hours of driving, the four of us and Oscar the cat arrived at our apartment complex. It was August 1977.

We settled into our three-bedroom Houston apartment and did the usual on-arrival task: purchasing the local newspaper to seek employment. We also wanted to establish connection with the local chapter of the Osteogenesis Imperfecta Foundation to get information on how we could obtain an electric wheelchair for Stephen.

There was little we could do until we had some income and security in our lives. Our days were long and increasingly desperate as we waited for employment. I was mainly engaged in tutoring Stephen, although he was more often tutoring me, especially in all things mathematical.

In the small apartment, we placed Stephen's bed in front of a wall from where he could watch TV and see outside through a big window. Oscar the cat would sit on the window ledge gazing happily outside.

One day Stephen said to me, "Mum, the wall is moving." I realised that this is what happens when you stare at a wall for a long time. We were going stir crazy. Thank goodness Stephen's electric wheelchair arrived soon after.

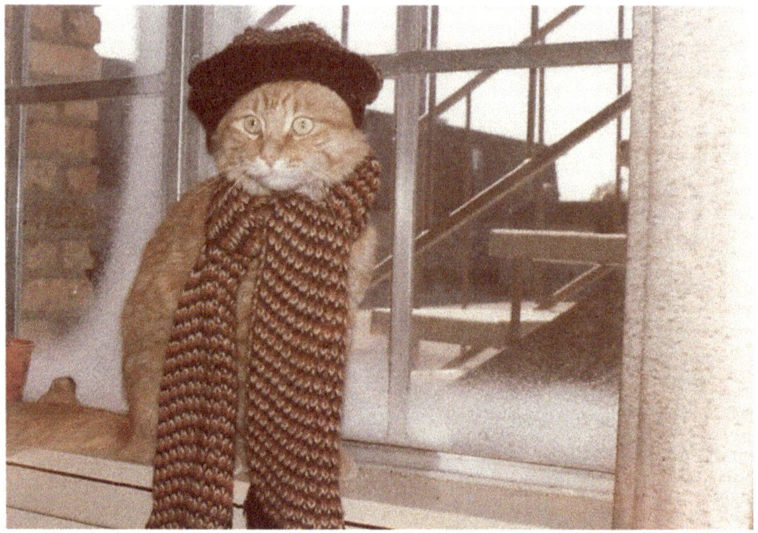

Oscar the cat

I set an appointment with the University of Houston for Stephen to take eligibility tests for attending classes. Stephen had successfully completed 11th Grade at home despite the ongoing challenge of physical pain and isolation. As 12th Grade wasn't available to be taught at home, he took the entrance exam for the University of Houston instead, achieving a very high score and qualifying to attend their classes.

After the test, Stephen went into the University garden and proceeded to doing figure eights and racing up and down the grounds at top speed. One young student walking with his friends said, "Hey, look at that kid having fun in a wheelchair." This behaviour was strange to them; being normal young men, they could not imagine anyone having that much fun in a wheelchair. But I knew very well that my boy was enjoying his newfound freedom in the best way after the confines of the apartment.

Ray was unfamiliar with metallurgical job opportunities in Houston and continued searching the daily papers for employment. After a few weeks, a small advertisement appeared seeking a Quality Control Manager for a local manufacturing facility. With little hope and no knowledge of the company or the product, Ray sent in his resumé.

Several days later the phone rang in our rented apartment and Ray was invited for an interview at a General Electric subsidiary. The directions to locate the factory were complicated, so much so that the person on the line indicated that if Ray arrived on time for the interview the job would most likely be his.

I wished Ray well the morning he set out for his interview. He returned some four hours later and described how he was interviewed by the Manager and escorted on a plant tour by the Chief Engineer. Then in the presence of them both, he was introduced to the Quality Control Foreman, who was an African American. This man bounded into the manager's office and shook Ray's hand firmly. The Manager and Engineer were intently watching Ray's reaction to the black man. Ray had greeted him in a sincerely welcoming manner without any racial prejudice. Once the foreman left, Ray was promptly hired at an attractive salary. Ray had been rewarded for his acceptance of others, regardless of race.

My relief at his employment was profound and we all celebrated our good fortune and marvelled at how far Ray's Diploma in Metallurgy from Perth Technical College had carried us though our life's journey. All those years of night school and studying had once again come to our rescue.

I was making Stephen comfortable for the night at about 11:00 PM. Ray had left a few hours earlier, and I was just mentioning to Stephen that he ought to be home by now when the phone rang.

"Harris County Precinct 6 Constable's Office here. We have your husband here for DUI. He ran into the back of a parked car and we are keeping him here till tomorrow."

I was furious. "Well, bloody well keep him there and rough him up a bit but don't break any bones."

"Yes, don't worry. It will cost you $500 to get him out of jail in the morning."

The next morning, I paid $500 to get Ray out. We could not afford losing so much money because of Ray's irresponsible behaviour. I supposed he was celebrating getting a job, but still that was no excuse.

Every day I searched for affordable housing, but with little knowledge of the Houston area this was no easy task. Then, three weeks into Ray's job, the Personnel Manager that Ray was chatting with informed him of a house for sale in the quiet wooded area in Cypress called Enchanted Valley, where he lived. It was close to the highway and only a 15 minutes' drive from work. With high hopes, we all loaded into our van and drove out to 12807 Blossomheath Drive, Cypress, Texas, the very next Saturday.

We instantly fell in love with the house, built on a half-acre block and surrounded by mature oak trees and home to sprightly squirrels. We checked our finances and found we were $500 short of the required deposit. Ray returned to work on Monday and reported this gloomy fact to the Personnel Manager.

"I can lend you that," was the immediate response. "Pay me back when you can afford it."

Ray was stunned that someone who had known him for only three weeks and who had only spoken to him to record his personal details would so generously offer to lend him $500 to buy a house! Ray vowed to repay the loan from his next pay, and we excitedly signed the necessary papers, bought our little piece of Texas and moved into our house in March 1978. The loan was duly repaid from the next paycheque and we were now settling into our new home.

Oscar the cat settled in immediately. It was a cat's paradise – a large forest backyard with tall American oak trees all around and little squirrels leaping from tree to tree. They were great entertainment for us. One day while having breakfast we saw a squirrel miss a branch and fall to the ground. We raced outside to help but the poor little squirrel was dead.

Animals were always great company for Stephen, as their soothing presence took his mind off his pain. I quickly acquired a beautiful tan crossed Labrador puppy and named her Mandy. Oscar and Mandy became firm friends. They romped and played together in the house and garden till both were exhausted, and then they would sleep together till their next game.

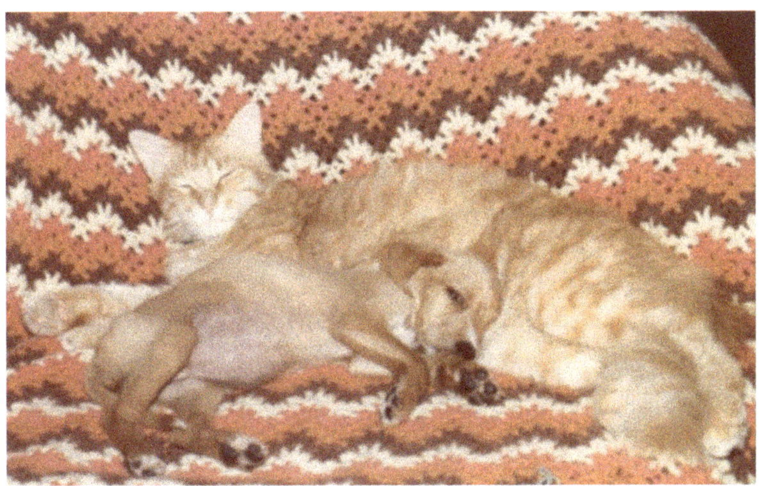

Good mates Oscar and Mandy

Houston was a great city for a variety of shows. Stephen had heard on the radio of a band called The Cars that would be playing at Houston Music Hall on June 21, 1979. He had never been to a live concert. He was so excited. The music and his heart beat together. A week later on June 28, we took him to see another band called Cheap Trick playing at the Houston Coliseum. Cheap Trick invited Stephen backstage, much to his delight. He impressed the band members with his knowledge of music and their songs. These concerts with loud music and lights radiating all around were a great stimulant for him and kept him in good spirits. The concerts really did him a world of good, and our hearts too seeing his happy face.

We took Stephen to four rock concerts just days apart. We saw a British band, The Fabulous Poodles. He was greatly amused by their hit Bionic Man. I think he imagined himself one day with bionic limbs replacing his own. He saw his favourite American bands, Tom Petty and the Heartbreakers, and Neil Diamond's hit, Hot August Night, our favourite.

The highlight of these concerts was The Hounds. The band's drummer jumped down from the stage and ran around like a lunatic everywhere, banging his drumsticks on the floor, making Stephen laugh so hard we were anxious he might crack a rib. Luckily, he didn't, and it did us good to see him enjoying himself so much. The band invited us backstage where the drummer gifted Stephen his drumsticks. Stephen cherished the drumsticks and kept them in a prized place all his life.

Stephen loved the sounds of the synthesizer keyboard. He spoke with the keyboard player John Hunter and over the years Stephen acquired over a dozen keyboards. The band was impressed with Stephen's knowledge of their music and treated him with great respect.

One night, after coming home from one of these concerts and turning on the TV, we found a show that caught Stephen's attention. Well, we all thought it was funny and bizarre. The show was called Monty Python's Flying Circus and the skit playing was 'the silly twit race'. We all laughed so hard that we had tears running down our cheeks. We never missed an episode after that. Stephen would recite every show word-for-word. His talent for mimicry always kept us and everyone laughing. His favourite accents to mimic were English, American, German and Texan.

15

Houston

One of the highlights of our time in Houston, Texas, was the chance to explore the home of NASA and the Johnson Space Centre. It was ten years since we had explored The Redstone Arsenal while living in Huntsville, Alabama.

Stephen, now a young man, gazed in awe from his electric wheelchair as he meandered through all the exhibits. The most interesting was the Apollo 11 command module. It was evident from the outside that it had been on fire while entering the earth's atmosphere. Inside the module was the incredibly small space that had housed three astronauts: Neil Armstrong, Buzz Aldrin and Michael Collins.

We saw Mission Control Centre. We recalled watching the moon landing on TV in Huntsville, Alabama, and hearing those now famous words spoken by Neil Armstrong: "Houston, Tranquillity Base here, the Eagle has landed."

Perhaps the most exciting incident relating to space happened on one particular day while driving down the freeway. Suddenly, Stephen shouted, "Look, look!"

Stephen, our little navigator, had spotted a magnificent sight. As we passed the main 610 highway ring road junctions, to our amazement, off to our left appeared a Jumbo 747 with a space shuttle attached to its back, obviously heading to the Ellington Air Force Base not far from Houston. We were driving parallel to the Jumbo and kept abreast of the plane for a good 4-5 minutes. We were enthralled at this impressive sight. Most people only saw this event on the news, so we considered ourselves incredibly lucky to have witnessed this spectacular sight. Naturally, this was a memory that stayed with Stephen all his life, and his model of the space shuttle pick-a-back on the 747 was among his favourites.

Ray's services, by then, were in demand at several locations, which involved lots of interstate travel. I was left to cope with running the house, home schooling Stephen and dealing with emergencies as they arose. Stephen often had many fractures at the same time, and trying to keep it all together, while Ray barely seemed to be home, became a bit much for me. I found myself becoming depressed.

Once, after I had readied Stephen for the day, I went back to bed feeling sad and tired of the constant struggles of my life. Stephen, sensing there was something wrong, came to my bedroom door in his wheelchair and asked, "What's the matter Mum?"

I looked up at him. "I feel so sad. I just can't get out of bed."

"You know what I do when I get like that, Mum?"

"No, what do you do?"

"I sing a song over and over in my head," he replied.

I looked at my boy smiling in his wheelchair. He couldn't walk, he had painful bones; he was practically stuck in his wheelchair.

I felt ashamed. I jumped out of bed and another miracle occurred as all the sadness and emptiness I had been feeling left me. I thought of the many times I had saved my dear boy from multiple disasters; here he was now, saving me this time.

Our neighbours on either side were as helpful as they were diverse.

On the right side of our house lived Syble and Jeff; they had two sons, Jeffrey Jnr and Johnnie, and a daughter, Janie. There was a vacant lot between our two houses. One day, I walked across the lot, knocked on their door and introduced myself. I explained that my husband had to suddenly go on a business trip, and I needed help to get my disabled son Stephen to the bathroom.

"No problem," Syble said. "I have two strong teenage boys here to help you."

The boys quickly became great friends with Stephen and when not in school, they would play together with Stephen's slot cars and track. Janie was adorable and just like a daughter to me. Syble and I clicked immediately and became firm friends, sharing our troubles daily at 4:00 PM over a bottle of wine.

To our left lived Hilda and Alfredo, who were from Cartagena, Columbia. We exchanged key words in English and Spanish in order to communicate. Their children, a boy and a girl, were learning English in school; they acted as interpreters whenever the adults were floundering because of their limited vocabularies.

To help Stephen's therapy, we built an insect proof enclosure on the concreted area at the rear of our house and installed a spa bath with eight persons' seating capacity. Alfredo, a carpenter by trade, offered to install the spa inside a cedar wood structure. The end result was very professional and pleasing to the eye. We planted all manner of plants in pots and spread them around the area. The bougainvillea and ferns gave the area a distinct tropical flavour. We built removable frames covered in plastic film which we attached in wintertime, and since the clothes dryer exhaust emptied into this area it was kept warm even on the coldest night. Word spread around the neighbourhood and soon we were welcoming newcomers to meet 'the Australians' and share our gas heated spa.

We made new friends in addition to our neighbours. Shirley and Bob with their son Richard and three daughters, Michelle, Kelly, and Jennifer, and Angela and John with their children Andrea and Richard. Through Angela, I obtained a secretarial position with her boss Paul. We became close friends with Paul and his wife Louise all enriching our lives and Stephen's. Many happy hours were spent around our barbecue and in the spa. Monday night football required moving the TV into the patio, where we watched many games from the spa.

Not long after the spa was put in, Ray got up on the roof to add some finishing touches. He put his foot on one of the enclosure rafters and, with a loud crack and bang, fell through onto the cement below. He sustained some deep scratches to his face but escaped any broken bones. Stephen and I were shocked at first, but when we saw him get up from the floor only shaken a bit, we laughed and were very relieved he had not broken a bone.

The spa was beneficial to Stephen as it allowed him greater freedom of movement in a semi weightless condition. Stephen improved physically, and visits to the Shriners Hospital ceased. It was unfortunate that the many surgical operations he had endured provided no lasting relief or improvement to his condition. He still suffered fractures to his collar bones, ribs, legs and arms. They were generally minor stress fractures but still very painful. Our expertise in applying plaster reinforcements was normally enough to avoid the trauma of X-rays and the accompanying breaks from being lifted onto X-ray tables.

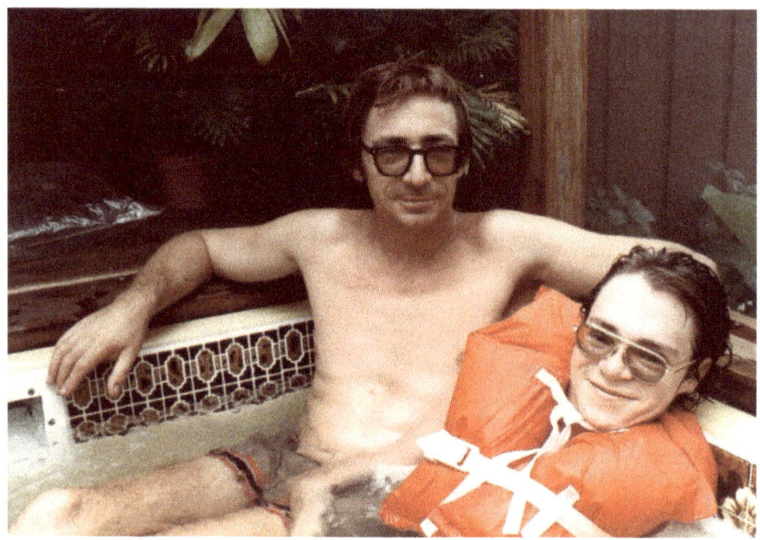

Stephen and Ray in the spa

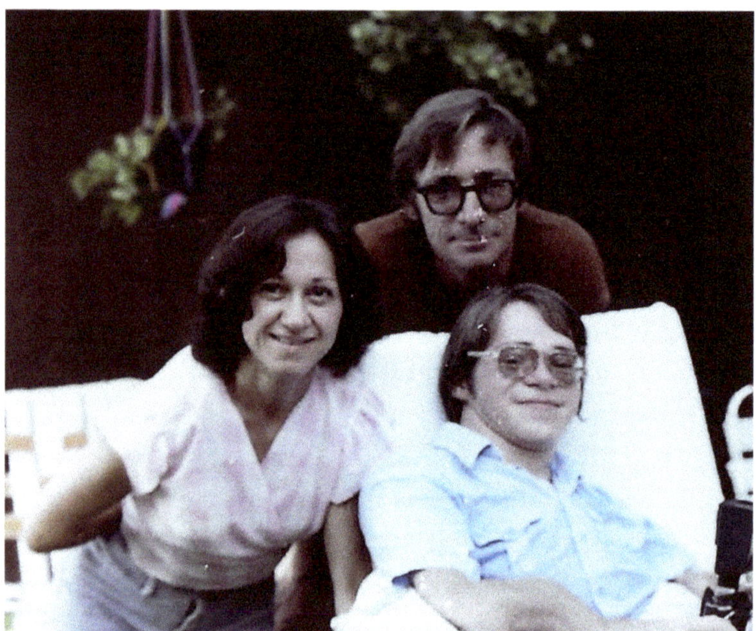

Me, Ray and Stephen in the patio

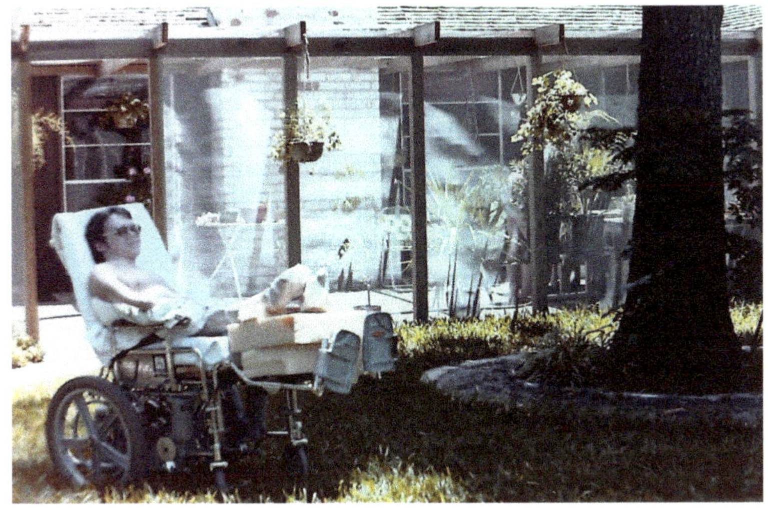

Stephen outside the spa

Stephen's new friends were accepting of his lack of physical mobility. They formed lasting friendships and were great company for each other. His best friend Richard, just a few years younger than Stephen, would play for hours with Stephen's slot cars. They would laugh uproariously while purposely crashing the cars, while I always kept a good supply of snacks and Coke.

I was giving Stephen a wash one morning as he lay in bed when the doorbell rang. I rushed to the door to see two Jehovah's standing with religious booklets in hand.

"I can't talk now. I am in the middle of helping my sick son," I said politely.

"We just want to read you something," they replied.

I immediately saw red. I recalled hearing about a little girl with pneumonia who had died after being pushed around all day at a Jehovah's convention, when the parents should have taken her to a doctor. The two men at the door did not show any concern for me and my predicament, nor did they offer to help. They were only interested in lecturing me about something in their brochure or selling me their booklet.

They said that God speaks to them all the time. I asked them if they had a disabled child, which they did not. I then asked them why God talks to them and not to me, when I have begged and pleaded for God to talk to me or guide me with my dilemmas. To that, they did not have an answer, so I bid them good day and shut the door, thinking how religion can blind one to reality.

In early February of 1980, Ray's mother came from Australia for another holiday. We showed her the many beautiful southern style homes in Houston, and again toured the Alamo and the Riverwalk in San Antonio. She enjoyed a social life of dinners and barbeques with our American friends and their families.

Stephen fell into a very dark mood in the beginning of March 1980. Even though we had made many aspects of Stephen's life enjoyable to the best of our abilities, he became depressed and did not enjoy listening to his music, which was most unusual. When I look back now, I see that the events unfolding in his life at the time were the cause of his depression. Stephen needed music, friends and intellectual stimulation as each had a direct influence on his mood and wellbeing.

His friends could not always come to visit each day due to school and their other interests. It was suggested by the Pastor at our church that being a carer for Stephen would be good for a young man he knew to get his mind off his own troubles and also would-be good company for Stephen. After less than a week, however, it became evident the young man selected was too immature and selfish and didn't want to work. Stephen, who had been excited at the thought of making a new friend, was extremely disappointed when this arrangement did not work out.

A huge burden for Stephen was he never wanted to worry us about his physical pain. If he experienced a stress fracture, he would go to great lengths to avoid troubling us with it. I thought back to my own childhood battles with OI and realised he was just like me; he did not want to upset his mother.

Not knowing what was going to happen to him in the future with his health left him at loose ends. Although we were committed to providing for Stephen, he still worried that he would be unemployable in the future. He felt he had no friends and no life. The frequent absence of Ray, who had always been a major source of support and intellectual stimulation to Stephen and me, contributed to our loneliness.

Stephen would lay awake at night, and I could not sleep either. One night, I got up and heard Stephen saying over and over, while wringing his hands. "Hold on. You're going to be all right."

I spoke softly to him. "What's the matter, fella?"

"I saw myself looking down on myself, and I think I want to die."

I was horrified. "No, no, no, you don't won't to die!"

"How do you know?"

"Well, because you are telling yourself to hold on over and over, and that means you do not want to die," I said, struggling to hide my tears.

He considered that for a moment and murmured in agreement. He was relieved, and I felt relieved too.

I was amazed at his out-of-body experience. I had heard of this phenomenon. From what I have read, Stephen's poor mental state and deprivation of sleep, together with his anxiety and depression, could have contributed to his experience.

Ray's mother was leaving to go back to Australia. On the way home after dropping her at the airport, we thought it best to take Stephen to the Hermann Hospital in Houston for an assessment of his condition. The hospital decided to admit Stephen. We explained to the nurses at length how to handle him and care for him, with his bone condition. He was distraught and miserable when we left him.

"Here we go again," I thought sadly on the way home without our poor boy.

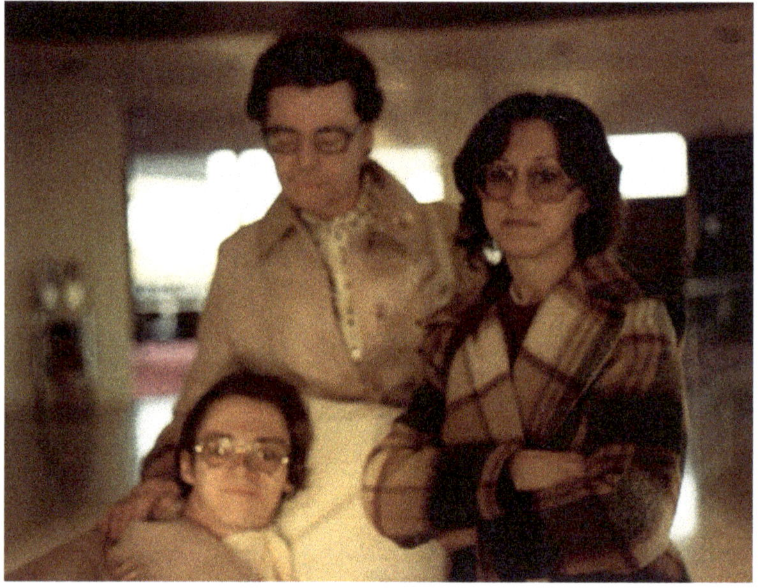

At Houston Airport, 1980

First thing the next morning, I called the doctors and asked how he was and if he had slept. They said that he had not, but there were six psychiatrists talking to him around the clock; he was quite okay and there was no need to worry. I called again the next morning and was overjoyed when they said that he had had 20 minutes of sleep. The least bit of good news always would give us new hope. The night after that he slept four hours. Relieved, we thought he was improving. The doctors then told us not to call. They said Stephen was less confused, he was going to be all right, and we should wait until he called us.

"What in the world is wrong with him?" I asked.

The doctor said, "Although he is 19 years old, he is going through a delayed adolescence or puberty blues. Most people go through puberty at 13, but his was delayed because of the lack of a normal life due to his condition."

I was relieved that this was the cause of his problem and that he wasn't losing his mind, despite the doctor's words not making any sense to me.

Finally, Stephen called us after a week. He was in a happy mood. He said he had met his roommate, a physicist, and they had talked about music till late at night. He said he had started playing piano in the recreation room at the hospital. The doctor said Stephen was now sleeping four to six hours a night. As he had plenty to occupy himself with in the day, they advised us not to visit for now.

After two weeks, Stephen phoned us again. He was angry that time, complaining about lack of hygiene. I think the nurses were cautious of handling him or showering him given his fragile bones. We decided to take him out to a movie for a change from his daily routine. We picked him up, but he was very unhappy on that day and argued with us over trivial things. When we took him back to the hospital, we spoke to the nurses and an orderly about the state he was in. They said he was discouraged by his physical condition and naturally, he was angry.

Stephen loved the social contact in his hospital ward and enjoyed talking with the doctors. And of course, there was the piano, which he loved to play with his one functioning right arm. He didn't want to come home.

Ray called him a week later and told him some news about John Lennon. Stephen said he was happy, he was having his breathing machine, and that his arm was feeling good.

Towards the end of March, Stephen was sleeping over six hours a night. The doctors told us that they were going to discharge him because he was well and having too much fun there.

With renewed hope, we looked forward to having our boy home again.

16

Houston Highs and Lows

Stephen came home from the hospital on April 4, 1980. He had been in the hospital five weeks. He slept well at first but within a few days he was unhappy again and not eating or sleeping.

One morning, just as I was about to wash his face, he slammed his fist down on the arm of his chair and yelled, "To think I am going to be in this wheelchair for the rest of my life."

I lost all hope then and did not know what to do or say to him. I guess I just carried on washing his face and hoped he would calm down.

I called a doctor who said Stephen should go into a nursing home. If that was his only solution, it was not going to eventuate. I would persevere in the face of whatever fate threw at us. I encouraged him to listen to music, as that lifted his spirits. It kept him going during the toughest of times.

The sun rose on December 8, 1980, like it does on any other day, but as we were watching the Monday night football game between the Miami Dolphins and the New England Patriots, the broadcast was interrupted with a news flash: "John Lennon murdered."

John Lennon had been returning home from his recording studio with his wife Yoko Ono when he was shot four times by a psychotic Beatles fan, Mark David Chapman, just as Lennon entered the archway outside his apartment in the Dakota building in New York City. Lennon was pronounced dead on arrival at Roosevelt Hospital.

We were stunned and found it difficult to believe what we had just heard. The Beatles had become so intrinsically woven into our lives that it felt like we had just lost a close family member. It was hard to go back to watching the game after this tragedy involving perhaps the most famous of all the Beatles.

For this shocking crime, Mark David Chapman was sentenced to life imprisonment. Sadly, we and the world were also sentenced to enduring the unnecessary loss of John Lennon and the gift of his music.

Trouble reared its head again. Stephen got bouts of colds, bronchitis and pneumonia which lasted off and on for over a year. It began with a high temperature and a bad cough. The doctor diagnosed bronchitis and prescribed antibiotics and inhalation therapy. His cough was so bad that I would place my hands gently on his ribs to help prevent fractures when he coughed. I watched him trying desperately not to cough, and it broke my heart. He suffered terribly when his ribs cracked under the strain.

After three weeks in this dreadful state, Stephen recovered. He then had a good nine months of home schooling, listening to music and racing remote controlled cars on his racetrack with a newfound friend, with only the occasional cold, headache or cough.

As was the usual pattern, good times did not last for Stephen. Pneumonia struck with the usual onset of symptoms and his health quickly deteriorated.

We rushed him down to Houston to see a doctor who prescribed a course of antibiotics. We then drove the 30 miles through peak hour traffic back home to Cypress. Stephen was extremely ill. I was frantic. I remembered a doctor telling me when Stephen was five years old that if he ever got pneumonia, "that would be it!"

What a nightmare of a trip home that was. I tried to help Stephen with his coughing by holding his ribs tightly and telling him over and over that he was going to be all right, while Ray tried his best to steer through the heavy Houston traffic. Finally, glad to get him home, we made him comfortable as best we could and never left his side.

At times, his cough would ease, allowing a brief respite, yet inevitably it would return. After each coughing attack and struggling not to break ribs while gasping for breath, Stephen was understandably exhausted and discouraged.

After a few days he started to brighten up. I made him chicken soup and healthy meals, sustaining him till the next crisis. He again had trouble breathing. His temperature rose quickly, followed by headache and sore throat, and once again pneumonia reared its ugly head. The doctors prescribed a different antibiotic, and I put him on a breathing machine every day to help clear his lungs. He bounced back for a few weeks, but then the whole ordeal began again.

Four difficult months were spent visiting doctors and trying different antibiotics with the usual inhalation therapy. We were desperately seeking relief for Stephen. Determined not to forget anything, I kept a written four-hourly record day and night of his medications and treatment and noted any improvement. Again, he would have a week's break in between, feeling better till the next onset.

Soon, pneumonia struck again. This time, in addition to the antibiotic, the doctor prescribed a marvellous medication called Theophylline. It aided the mechanics of pulmonary ventilation or breathing, which hastened his recovery. After the course, Stephen's health slowly improved and within two months his temperature stopped spiking and was back to normal.

Pharmaceutical medications may have saved Stephen's life, but music saved his spirit. Music helped Stephen express his emotions and offered an incredible source of enjoyment. It is a well-known fact that music is a great healer. It helps to reduce stress, decrease pain and boost immunity. These truths were well evidenced in Stephen's life. Music was like a set of working limbs for Stephen; it took him to places he couldn't go himself and introduced him to a whole new world.

During this time, Stephen's taste in music began to broaden. While convalescing, he listened to other bands as well as The Beatles and The Rolling Stones. We bought him a lightweight small keyboard that he could tolerate balancing across his lap for short periods. He quickly learned to play any tune by ear with his one good right hand.

Due to necessity, Ray purchased two aluminium motorcycle ramps, allowing Stephen to drive his wheelchair in and out of our Chevy van. This made transporting him to and from hospital and to doctor appointments much easier.

On one unforgettable day, I had just arrived home with Stephen from a routine doctor's visit. I jumped out of the van and proceeded to line Stephen's wheelchair up to the ramp. To my horror, I noticed as Stephen reversed that the front left wheel had twisted out of the ramp.

"Stop! The wheel has come out of the ramp!" I yelled.

I knew that if the wheelchair fell from the ramp, it would result in multiple fractures for Stephen – the last catastrophe he needed. I could not let this happen.

By placing my right leg on the step of the van and taking the weight of the wheelchair with my knee, I reached a long distance forward with my left hand to try to twist the wheel back into the ramp. I could hear Syble, my neighbour, talking from across the vacant lot. I tried to call her, but my voice was only a whisper. All my strength was being used to hold Stephen in his chair, while at the same time reaching desperately to put the wheel back into the ramp slot. Stephen remained calm, trying to guide me in this dreadful dilemma. He talked me through the whole ordeal and miraculously, I finally got the wheel into the slot and Stephen wheeled safely out of the van.

Gleefully, I thought of little me as Superwoman! God must have helped me do that! I could not believe that I had managed this seemingly impossible feat of strength. Where I got the strength from, I have never known. I just believed I could do it, and I did.

As Stephen's health improved, he further mastered his wheelchair, allowing him to venture around the neighbourhood, meet new friends, and have more freedom to explore. The Houston summers were hot with 100 percent humidity. I purchased a small used bike in good order. After dinner each night in the cool of the evening, Stephen and I would race each other around the block. Hilariously, Stephen in his wheelchair would beat me on my little bicycle. I would be shouting at him to slow down and be careful. It was always thrilling, risking the danger of anything happening, and then getting home safe. We had so much fun. We have so many happy memories of those days long ago.

Meanwhile, Ray was fascinated by his work duties as Quality Control Manager at the facility manufacturing Tungsten Carbide inserts for oil drilling and coal mining industries. He was surprised by the many facets of the manufacturing process that seemed so antiquated. Despite never having worked in the industry, he resolved to concentrate on bringing about changes that would streamline the process, save time and money, as well as improve the overall manufacturing efficiency.

Within a short time, my clever husband, having made several manufacturing improvements and been recognised by the Detroit head office for his contributions, was promoted to Senior Metallurgist. He was given carte blanche to pursue a wide-ranging suite of projects, not only for the Houston and Detroit plants but also encompassing work on artificial diamonds and other industries contained under the umbrella of General Electric.

Several months following his promotion, Ray came home and told me that a separate laboratory was being built within the Houston facility, furnished with state-of-the-art metallurgical equipment. Pride of place was reserved for the little sintering furnace that he had designed. It cost a sizeable sum of $300,000 and was only the size of a microwave oven. I was amazed at the cost, and Ray explained that the revolutionary feature of the furnace allowed cooling from 1,400 degrees centigrade to room temperature in just a few minutes. The standard furnaces of that time required 12 hours or more to cool down, due to the vacuum they contained. This aspect of Ray's invention revolutionised the construction of future industrial-scale furnaces and, in effect, doubled the sintering throughput. It all went over my head, of course, but Stephen could understand it all, and I happily furnished our house with the salary increment.

After Christmas and New Year 1981, Stephen became unhappy again. A math teacher was coming to tutor him, but it turned out Stephen was teaching him rather the other way around, so there was no stimulation for Stephen, which was disappointing. Moreover, as winter gave way to spring, both of Syble's boys took on jobs after school. Jeffrey was working at a gym and Johnny at a nearby supermarket. Richard, Stephen's slot car racing buddy, was spending time with his dad since his parents had split up. All of this added to Stephen's loneliness.

It would soon be Stephen's twenty-first birthday, and we thought we would take him home to Australia for a holiday to lift his mood.

I wrote a letter to the care facility for disabled children that Stephen had stayed in when we had been in Australia in 1974, asking them if they could care for him again while we paid visits to family and friends. Unfortunately, they did not have a vacancy, but said Stephen could sleep in his reclining wheelchair until a bed became available. It was good to learn that most of his carers and mates were still there even after seven years, which would make his situation more comfortable.

Ray arranged for two weeks' leave from his work and booked the air tickets. He sorted the transportation of Stephen's wheelchair and its revolutionary sealed batteries. We were all set to be off to the airport for our trip home to Australia via San Francisco, Hawaii and Sydney. Saying goodbye to his friends and his beloved pets Oscar and Mandy did not bode well, however, for Stephen getting over his gloom.

We had arranged to stay overnight in Sydney with some family friends that we had not seen for many years. We had a good flight. Stephen was thrilled to be flying again, and was most excited with the take-offs and landings. He was awake most of the time, enjoying looking out the small window even when there was nothing to see. We relished in his joyfulness thinking we were doing the right thing for him.

We arrived in Sydney on time to glorious autumn weather. After collecting Stephen's wheelchair and our luggage, we were immediately whisked off to a backyard barbecue. Stephen's wheelchair was a great topic of conversation due to its innovative manoeuvrability, and Stephen was only too happy to demonstrate its many capabilities.

After a very sound sleep, we accepted our host's offer of transport to the airport, where we boarded our flight for the final leg of our journey to Perth.

17

The Bird Has Flown

We arrived home in Perth to be met by Glasses Nana and my brother Tom, now home from his travels around America. They made the usual fuss of our little family, discussed current economic conditions in Australia and America, and made the usual enquiries as to when we were coming home to live. Seeing his relatives again certainly helped Stephen's disposition. He was the

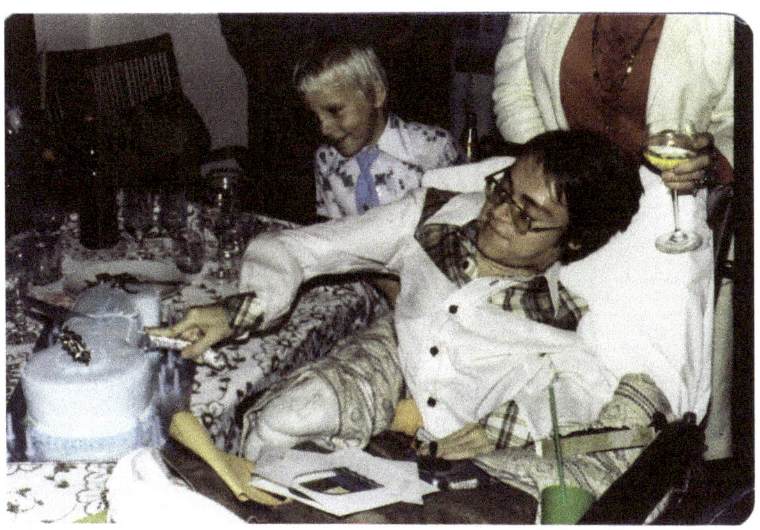

Stephen's twenty-first birthday, 26 April 1981, with his cousin Brendon

centre of attention as he held them spellbound with stories of his comings and goings in America. Stephen's twenty-first birthday was spent at Glasses Nana's house with family and friends. It was a wonderful day full of laughter.

After two weeks of rushing here, there and everywhere visiting family and friends, the time had come to fly back to America. The day before we were to leave, Stephen announced that he did not want to go back with us. He wanted to stay at the nursing home, where he had 24-hour care available to him and relatives in the same town. He felt it was a wise decision to stay, given his condition.

Whenever we had visited him at the nursing home, I had watched him enjoying the company of young men working as male carers who were going to university to study architecture or medicine, as well as some young men with muscular dystrophy whom Stephen had befriended. Altogether, they were a bunch of intellectuals thriving on conversations of all topics, which was stimulating to him. I could see why he did not want to come back with us to America; nevertheless, we were shocked at his decision.

The day came when we had say goodbye and return to America for Ray's work. I was terribly upset about travelling back to America without Stephen. My face was swollen from crying when we landed in Hawaii. Immigration hardly recognised me from my passport photo. Ray briefly explained we had to leave our disabled son back in Australia.

I hated the fact that we would not be with him to protect him from the evils of the world. I was overwhelmed at his surprising decision to stay back and cope by himself with the battles we knew awaited him. My brave, soldier boy would have to battle on without us. We learned later that Stephen missed us terribly.

We would speak to him every Sunday evening, Perth time, from Houston. At first, he seemed to be coping well but soon depression set in once again. My family visited him often and my kind Aunt Peg, the matriarch of our family, even stayed overnight several times when Stephen was at his lowest, to give him support and encouragement. This was a great comfort for me. Every week Aunt Peg arranged for Stephen to visit her, my cousins and their children. These visits lifted his spirit. Also included was my mother, who was now living in a nursing home. Both Stephen and my mother, the Talking Nana, valued this weekly family get-together.

One reason for his depression was that the supervision staff at the nursing home insisted that he take his pain medication every four hours as prescribed, just like a metronome, even if his pain was tolerable. Stephen would telephone us, livid. He was having constant arguments with the staff about his pain medication.

"They won't let me take my pain pills in the way that works best for me," he'd tell us miserably.

Stephen wanted to manage his pain as per his own time scale and didn't want the medication controlling him. He wanted to regulate his dosage to just control his pain enough when he most needed it, in order to be able to do the things he enjoyed. He did not want to be constantly medicated to the point if he were sleeping and he twitched or moved the wrong way, it could cause a stress fracture. He wanted to just cover his pain and play his music or his keyboard. This was impossible if he was drowsy from the medication.

The pain-pills regime that was forced on him had no flexibility to cater to his individual needs. It was so cruel. They would not listen to him or me, insisting he take the medication like clockwork regardless of his needs. Stephen's situation was extremely upsetting, and we felt helpless being so far away. I pleaded with the staff; surely, they could turn a blind eye? But they stuck to the rules, proud of their rigidity and heartless inflexibility.

Meanwhile, life in America seemed empty and lacking in purpose with Stephen being so far away in a care facility in Australia. Our calls with Stephen would only add to our worries, as we had no control over the situation and felt helpless and dejected.

Ray was engaged in his work, which relieved much of his anxiety, but another blow was waiting in the wings. Despite having made advances in the processes employed at his workplace and attained the respect of Department Heads of other Divisions in the company, Ray was retrenched during a cost-cutting exercise in the oil industry downturn of that time. We were out of a job again. Since our good friends Paul and Louise had moved to Florida, I was also unemployed. I had worked as a secretary to Paul in a big international company before, but when Paul was asked to relocate his office to another State, he had opted for voluntary retirement. This only served to compound my grief at having left Stephen behind, even though he was adamant about staying and had mostly settled in well.

As fate would have it, Ray was contacted by an Australian entrepreneur who had designed and was manufacturing some water sports equipment. He was coming to America to sign a contract with an American company to manufacture his equipment and, via a mutual friend, had arranged to stay with us for a few days. On paper, the equipment looked like a real money spinner, catering to the ever-increasing tourist trade. Ray contacted Paul, who agreed to lend him $10,000 to buy ten 'water bikes' to be shipped from Australia – the basis of a brave new adventure.

Ray flew to Honolulu, Hawaii, and walked along Waikiki beach asking various concessionaires if they would rent him some space on the beach to conduct his business. He was met with a solid wall of resistance, but a passer-by directed him to the office of a local businessman who offered to rent him some beach area and a storage enclosure for $3,000 per month. When he asked about the nature of the business, Ray told him he was going to rent 'bikes' that you could ride on the water, charged at $10 for 30 minutes. The businessman was flabbergasted and told Ray he was mad; the existing beach vendors sold coconuts and outrigger canoe rides for $3 and hardly made a living.

Despite this grim warning, the partners persisted and as a consequence, Ray and I flew to Honolulu and rented an apartment for $400 per month. This was ideally situated, only five minutes' walk to the famous Waikiki Beach. We were excited about our new venture. Hawaii, which was situated at eight hours' flying time from both Sydney and Houston and had wonderful weather, was a dream location for us.

After a month's delay due to 'industrial action' on the wharves in Sydney, our equipment finally arrived. Ray hired a local young man to help him. We took delivery of the bikes at sundown at our rented storage facility. This again was ideally located right on the beach, surrounded by a high and lockable wrought iron fence. Ray and his helper immediately assembled one bike and decided to try it out on the water. They paddled out about 50 yards from the beach and were having a great time. Looking shore-wards, they noticed a large crowd gathering at the shoreline, pointing and making remarks about the two heroes riding on water.

Adjacent to our storage, a well-known hotel had a restaurant with large plate-glass windows overlooking the beach. Ray noticed patrons lining up behind the glass, peering out the windows at this strange apparition: two people riding the gentle waters with minimum effort. The riders eventually came ashore, happy as can be and bubbling over with enthusiasm. They could not wait for the morning to assemble all the bikes and get into business.

Morning came. Ray, our helper and I were at our base early, and while they assembled the bikes, I set up our beach umbrella, card table and chair to begin rentals. I had rental agreements printed for insurance purposes which explained that if the renter was hurt in any way it was their fault and not ours! Each renter was to sign the form, which we kept it in a cardboard box until they returned.

The demand that first day outstripped the assembly line. I explained to those waiting that the cost was $10 per half-hour plus a $10 deposit, refundable on return of the bike. This was readily accepted and as the bikes became available, they were immediately rented. At the end of our first day, we had made $600! When we arrived home at our rented apartment, we sat on the bed and threw the money up in the air, laughing our heads off. We had never seen such an abundance of money for so little effort on our part. We had a lot of fun stacking the 'green backs' face up, which was much appreciated by the bank.

Next day, with all 10 bikes available, we made $1,100, and this flood of money kept coming over the days ahead. Even on our worst day, when it rained all day, we made $450.

The local bank we had joined would not deposit traveller's checks directly into our account, explaining that there was a three-week delay before the cash would be available. This was upsetting, but at the end of the first week, seeing how we were definitely in business, the bank relented and made the money instantly available. Ray would walk to deposit our takings at 5 o'clock every afternoon, except on Sundays, strolling along the beachfront with the money in a plastic bag, wearing our newly printed T-shirt and being warmly welcomed at the bank.

Our success created much envy among the local beach vendors. Resentment soon became evident. Our neighbouring vendor, a native Hawaiian who had initially been helpful, was soon treating us rather coolly.

One day, Ray noticed a disabled person sitting in his wheelchair, watching the bikes with great interest. Ray asked the young man if he would like a ride and the response was an eager "Yes!" Ray asked our neighbour, a strapping, big, healthy Hawaiian, if he would take the young man for a ride. It was agreed that they would stay away from the breaking waves some distance from shore. We seated the young man on board and tied his feet to the structure, as he had no control over his lower limbs, and off they went. Next thing we noticed, they were out riding the forbidden waves and when they finally returned, the look on their faces was priceless. Both agreed it was the best fun they had had in ages.

Next day, 54 wheelchair-bound people visited the beach, as part of some convention sponsored by a charitable group. All of them, with the help of volunteers, had a ride for free. On that day we made no money, but a feeling of contentment persisted as we had added tremendous joy, if only for one day, to the lives of these people. We were thrilled to know that they would remember their half hour of total freedom for the rest of their lives.

We settled into a daily regime of being on the beach at 7:00 AM. Ray would rake our area of the beach, removing any rubbish the tourists had left behind. It was a point of pride that the first beachgoers would see the newly raked beach and were aware that someone cared for the comfort of tourists. In the meantime, I would set up our little business area and Ray and his helper would bring the bikes out of the enclosure ready for business, which started as soon as the bikes hit the sand.

Everyone who rode the bikes had a great time, and we had many repeat customers. We met people from all over the world and everyone had an interesting story to tell. Hawaii at that time was the 'in' place, but many European tourists indicated that Maldives was gaining in popularity and would most likely be their next vacation destination.

We were making so much money that we attracted a local standover gang who wanted to share our takings on a 50:50 basis. One day there appeared a gentleman dressed immaculately in a tailor-made suit and expensive Italian shoes, who invited Ray into the adjacent building 'for a chat'.

A few minutes later I looked through the big glass windows and saw this man swinging a Hawaiian 'koa' fighting stick within a whisker of Ray's nose! The man was making Ray an offer he assumed Ray would be unable to refuse. But Ray deemed the proposal too tiresome and asked to be excused to return to the beach. The man was dumbfounded at this, and from then on mysterious happenings occurred, all aimed at intimidating us to sell 50% of our business to the standover merchants for $1.

To illustrate the idiocy of this proposal, Ray determined that we would not open for business the next day. We took time off to go shopping and generally relax while people on the beach wondered where we were. The following morning, the man arrived and enquired as to what was going on and Ray held out his empty hand and said, "Here's your share of yesterday's takings: zero!"

After that, bloodstained towels and packages of human excrement began appearing outside our apartment door. Objects would fall from the upper levels of the beachfront building, narrowly missing me as I sat on my chair renting out the bikes. After these dastardly episodes I became ill with anxiety and feared for our lives.

After two and a half months of Hawaiian paradise and $1,000-a-day money flow, the bikes started to break down and surprisingly, the standover man helped repair them! Ray knew that the bikes were close to collapsing totally and agreed to sell the business for $2,000, instructing the man to be at our bank at 9:00 AM the following morning with a cheque. Once this was done and the money safely put in the bank, we went on a tour of the USS Arizona Memorial at Pearl Harbor. We hired a car and drove all around the Island of Oahu, which helped me to relax a little.

After a few days, we went back to the beach and we were approached by the new owner, who said, "All your bikes have broken down!"

Ray replied, "They are your bikes now, but I will buy them back for $1,000 and fix them properly."

We passed over a cheque for the purchase price. We then rented whatever bikes we could while Ray carried out repairs. This went on for a few days until the standover man returned, demanding, "We want our bikes back!"

Ray pointed out that they were our bikes now, and a further $2,000 would be required to change ownership back to the standover man. This made him truly mad, but it was agreed that they would meet at 11:00 AM at the bank the next morning and seal the deal.

That night we packed our bags and transferred all our funds to Houston, ready for instant departure. Next morning, with the cheque cashed, we headed for the airport and secured our seats on a flight to Houston. We could see the man and his standover collaborators running through the various arms of the airport, looking for the 'Haoles' (white people) who had outsmarted a bunch of hooligans, thus ending our dream of 'working' midway between our homeland, Australia, and our residence in Houston, Texas.

18

More Adventures

Having fled Hawaii just ahead of our Mafia type pursuers, we returned to our house in Houston. Ray had little prospect of finding a metallurgical position as the economy was still in a downturn. We had enjoyed our time in Hawaii so much that we decided to approach a prominent lawyer who might be interested in funding a larger operation in the Caribbean Sea. He approved our proposal and arranged funding from a number of his clients.

This marked the start of our next new adventure. New bikes were purchased from the American manufacturer, and we were granted exclusive rights to the entire Caribbean Sea area, including all the islands of the West Indies and the east coast of Mexico. Ray and I were enthusiastic at this turn of events and began scouting for concessionaires and locations to operate the bikes.

Initially we headed to Nassau, the capital city of the Commonwealth of Bahamas which is made up of 700 islands. Discovered by Christopher Columbus in 1492, the clear blue seas were named 'Baja Mar' which is Spanish for shallow seas, and the islands later came to be known as 'Bahamas'. Nassau in the 1600s was the home of Blackbeard, a notorious pirate, and the well he drew his water from has been preserved to this day. We were impressed by the colourful Changing of the Guard ceremony which took place at noon on Saturdays, thus preserving the nation's British heritage. Nassau was also a popular cruise ship destination on Paradise Island, just a short distance away and connected by a causeway.

We contracted a well-established water sports company with a highly visible site on a beautiful beach to be our first concessionaires, and then headed to a bank owned by a British celebrity to open an account in this beautiful tax-free island. The celebrity had risen from a humble beginning to achieve millionaire status, eventually owning elite businessmen's clubs in London, America and several Caribbean Islands.

Having established our initial site and completed all the business requirements, we returned to Houston and placed our initial order for equipment. The five water bikes that arrived in Nassau were popular as soon as they were assembled, and we had high hopes for the success of this venture.

Our next location was to be established in the lush green island of Jamaica. We flew into Montego Bay and drove our hired car to the resort town of Ocho Rios, an up-and-coming tourist area with two large hotels on the beach and little in the way of water sports or recreational activities. We contacted a local sportsman who pledged loyalty and came with good references, to operate the concession. Ultimately, though, he proved a poor choice and stole most of our income; but these were heady days when everything looked rosy.

While waiting for our equipment to arrive in the port of Kingston, we took a tour of the island. We headed towards Port Antonio to fulfil my lifelong dream of visiting the estate of the famous Australian movie star, Errol Flynn.

Along the way we visited the magnificent Trident Hotel, where it was rumoured that Flynn's wife, Patrice Wymore, ran a little boutique. It was a very glamorous hotel in a pretty oceanside location with gold-rimmed China and gold-plated cutlery set upon tables. We did not get to meet Ms Wymore, so we pressed on to Port Antonio proper and found our way to a hilltop residence featuring a large billboard bearing the inscription: ERROL FLYNN ESTATES.

Unbelievable! Here I was so far from home in Western Australia, looking at the home of my idol, Errol Flynn, who had died in 1959 at the tender age of 50. As we stood at the swing gate at the farm entrance, we noticed a Jamaican man leading a fine-looking horse. He approached us and we immediately started to bombard him with questions about his years of service for Errol Flynn, the great man. He was pleasant and warm in nature and had us enthralled with the tales of his adventures and eventually allowed me to pat the horse and get on its back. We were captivated by the view from the estate, looking upon 2,000 acres of lush farmland and horse pasture.

The other area we visited was the beach at Negril, Rose Hall, where we were enthralled with tales of witchcraft and murders. All the while we detected a faint odour of marijuana, or 'ganja' as it is known in Jamaica, wafting through the air. Soon, we were revelling in white water rafting on the White River, then climbing up Dunn's River Falls, exploring the sights and sounds, especially Reggae music, until it was finally time to collect our cargo from Kingston. We drove through Fern Tree Gully, through thick jungle and over mountains and streams to Kingston and back. We were delighted with the most beautiful island of the Caribbean.

In two days, we set up the bike business in Ocho Rios and with many reassurances from our new best friend, headed back to 'Mobay' to fly back to our home in Houston.

After a brief rest, we were told of a scuba diving business in Cozumel, Mexico, which had made enquiries regarding operating some water bikes. Ray obtained the necessary visas and set out to Mexico with an official-looking briefcase, to be met at the airport by the Dive Shop owner named Juan.

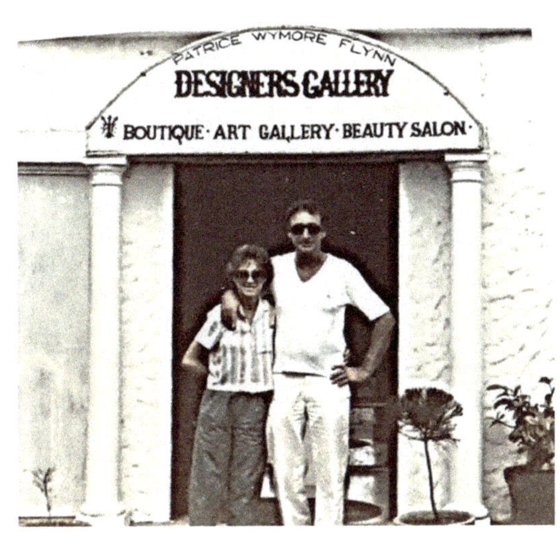

Us at Patrice Wymore Boutique

The little airport was busy with passengers who had arrived on the plane and those who were waiting to board the same plane. Eventually, only two people were left: Ray with his briefcase and a handsome Mexican man wearing swimming trunks and sandals. He approached Ray with a smile and said, "You should have recognised me, I'm the only one here wearing trunks, because it's how I earn my living." They departed to Juan's house and after many beers, agreed upon a verbal contract. This was the first of many visits, and a great friendship developed between us and his family.

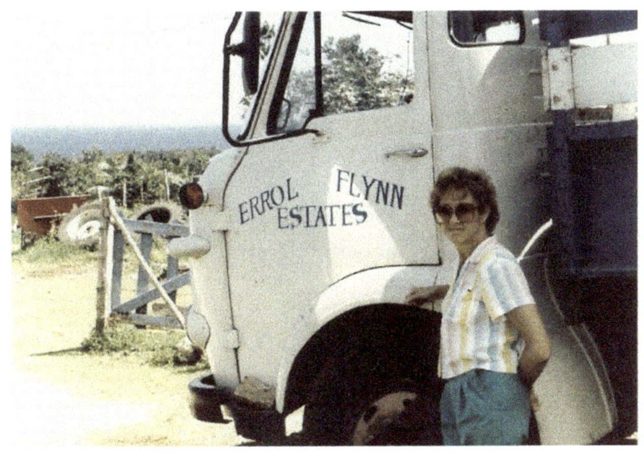

Me with Errol Flynn's truck

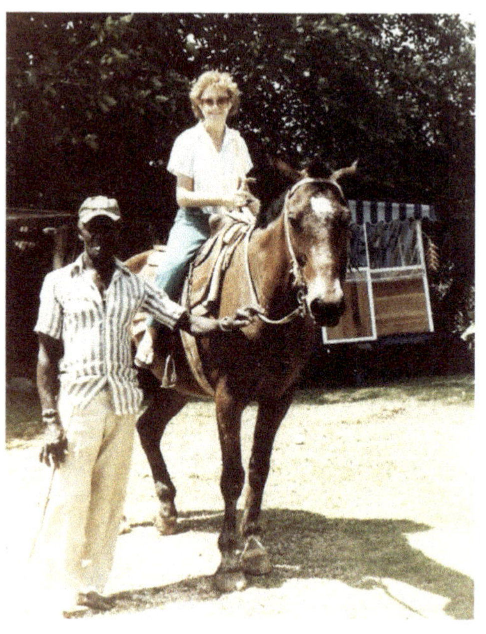

Jamaican man and me on Errol Flynn's horse

Once the bikes were imported, Ray and I flew to Cozumel to assemble the equipment and get the business started. We were entertained by our new partner and his wife Rosa and treated to a tour of the island.

We were fascinated by the local Mayan ruins and an aeroplane on the ocean floor in the harbour. The water was so clear, you could see all the individual rivets in the wings, yet the plane was in water metres deep. Our friend Juan in Cozumel was well known in the diving fraternity, and Ray's attendance at diving shows with him

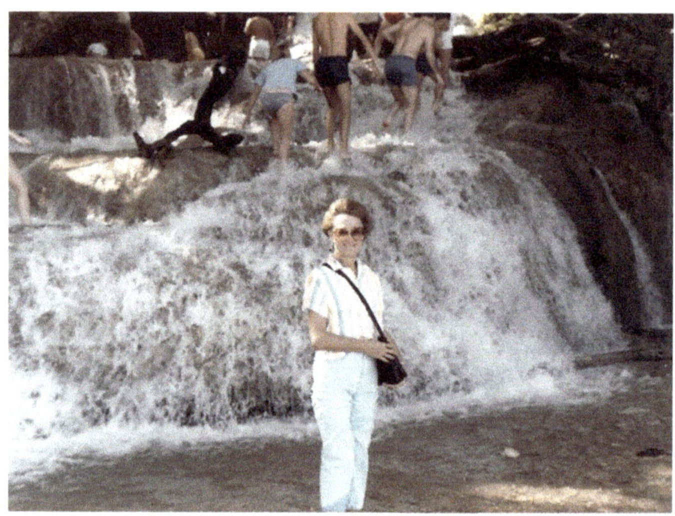

Me at Dunn River Falls

led to more opportunities to place the bikes. This resulted in travel to exotic locations throughout the Caribbean, and soon Ray's passport was full of stamps to the Cayman Islands, Barbados, Turks and Caicos, Jamaica, Trinidad and Tobago, the U.S. Virgin Islands of St. John and St. Croix, Charlotte Amalie in the British Virgin Islands, Puerto Rico, Costa Rico and various smaller locations throughout the Bahamas.

In time, counterfeit bikes began to appear on several beaches. We learned that a prior workmate of Ray's had joined forces with a slick salesman, and together they had enrolled some investors to manufacture crude imitations of the bikes. The investors contacted Ray, complaining that they did not know how many bikes they owned or where they were located. They had received no return on their investment and were keen for Ray to find the bikes and operate them in Galveston, Texas.

This mildly appealed to Ray, as he considered he had been double-crossed by the promoters due to Ray's allegiance to the original licensed manufacturer. He contacted a former employee from Hawaii who had returned to the U.S. after the Hawaiian closure, and together they set about scouting Florida beaches and recording the serial numbers of the counterfeit bikes. The supposed 'owners' each signed a document showing that they owned all the bikes discovered on the various beaches.

With a sense of adventure, Ray and Tom, his ex-workmate from Hawaii, set off for the beaches in Florida and mapped out a hit-and-run strategy for removing the counterfeit bikes. With a large removal truck, they approached one site and started loading the equipment. The operator protested strongly and called the police, who appeared in a dramatic blaze of sirens and flashing lights. Ray showed them the papers of dubious legality, and the police confirmed that the removal could go ahead.

These operations were repeated in various locations, much to the frustration of the clandestine promoters. Despite their endeavours, the Florida beaches were cleaned of fake bikes and our two daring heroes returned to Houston. Some of the bikes that were captured were placed in Galveston, about an hour from Houston, and others returned to their owners throughout Texas.

Meanwhile, all was not well in the Caribbean. The only locations forwarding any revenues to us were Nassau and Cozumel, together with a pittance from Jamaica. Ray flew to Jamaica unannounced and spent a day watching the rental operation from a discreet location, only to learn that the business was, in fact, running well and most of the bikes were rented all the time.

At the end of the day, Ray approached his so-called friend-in-charge and demanded the day's takings of about $1,100. The operator begged forgiveness and promised to send all the moneys owed within the week. Ray was not convinced and placed the bikes in charge of an opposition beach operator adjacent to our original location. This added insult to injury to our ex-concessionaire, who screamed obscenities until the police removed him. An improved income returned for a short time, and then the equipment was moved to a different location. We never received another penny or knew where our equipment was being rented.

Ray and Tom continued to operate in Galveston on the weekends to provide some income. The lack of money from other locations, coupled with the expense of airfares in search of missing revenues, placed a huge strain on my mental wellbeing.

We often visited Australia to see Stephen at the nursing home. When in America, we made numerous phone calls to talk to him and ensure he was okay. On each trip home, we would bring musical equipment that Stephen needed. We brought power converters, transformers, CD players, an amplifier, and various items to be set up in his room where he could play his music to his heart's content.

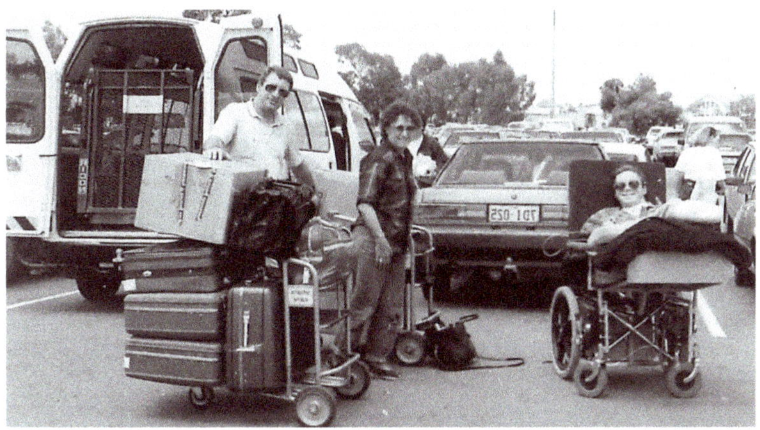

Steve meeting us with his music gear

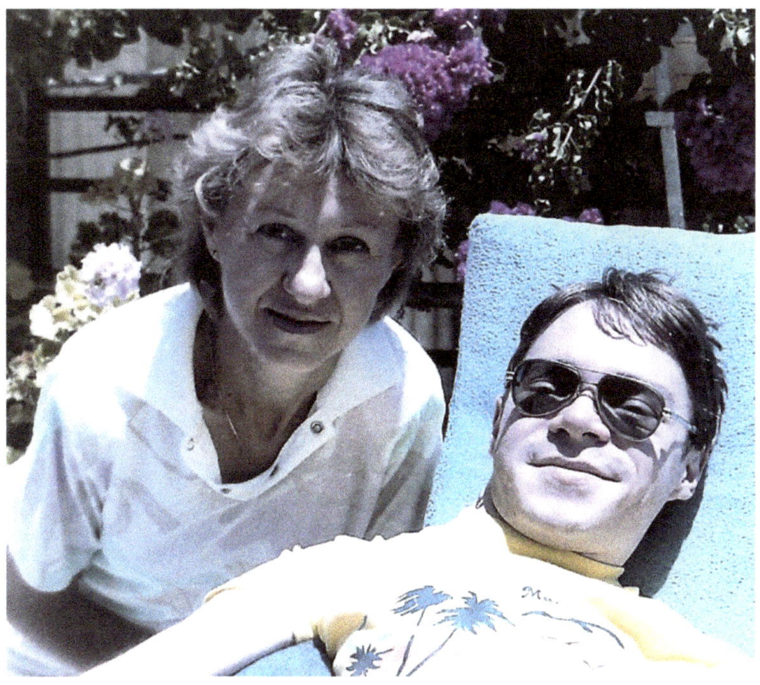

Visiting Stephen

It was a relief seeing Stephen happy and involved in various activities. I was more at ease returning to America knowing he was in a better place in Australia with many new friends and in good care.

On trips to and from Australia to visit Stephen, we toured many places. We saw the Statue of Christ the Redeemer in Rio, Brazil, as well as Iguazu Falls, the largest waterfall system in the world. We went boat sailing on the Amazon River to Manaus. We saw Eva Peron's Tomb in La Recoleta Cemetery in Buenos Aires, and also encountered Argentinian cowboys, Gauchos, where we spent a wonderful day being entertained with barbecues and horses.

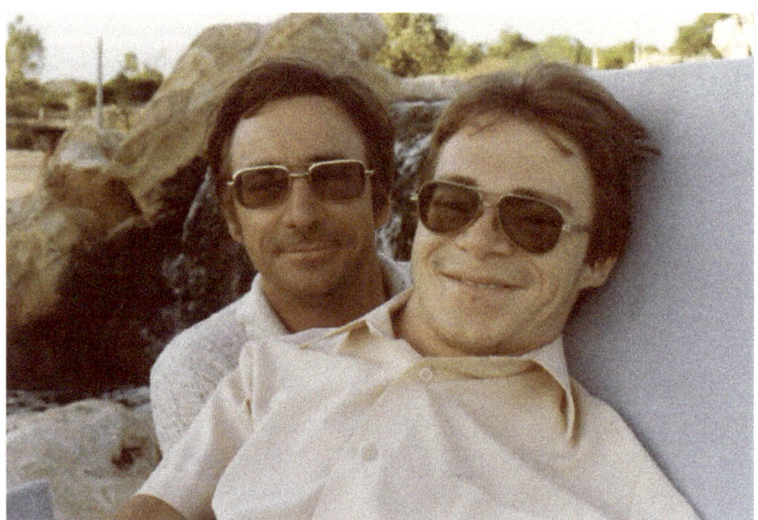

Visiting Stephen

One night, after settling back in our home in America, I woke up at 4:30 AM thinking about my mother. Just then, I received a phone call from my brother telling me that our mother had died. I lay in bed for hours thinking about all the beautiful words she had spoken to me and all the things she had done in her life.

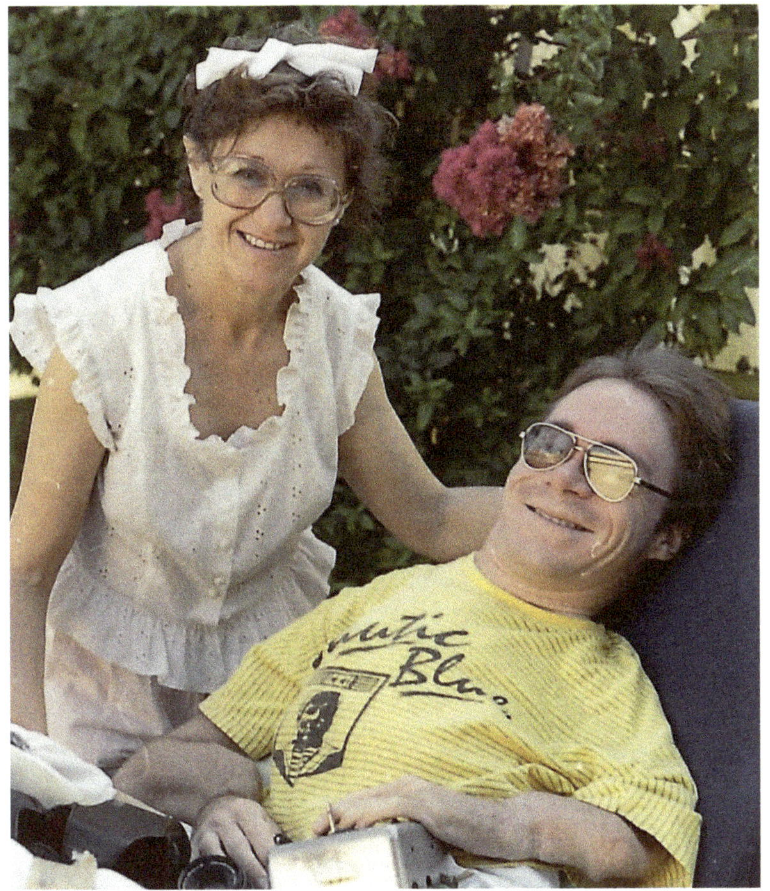

Visiting Stephen

The last time I had seen my mother on our previous trip to Australia, she had been lying quietly in bed while I talked to her. She did not answer me, except when I asked her about my brother Tom. She raised her head then and replied, "Good," before sinking into silence again. Heartbroken, I had put my head down beside her on her bed and cried, realising intuitively that I may never see her again. She had put her hand lovingly on my head as I wept. When I was walking out of her room, a nurse noted my tears and sadness and remarked kindly, "We all lose our mums, love!"

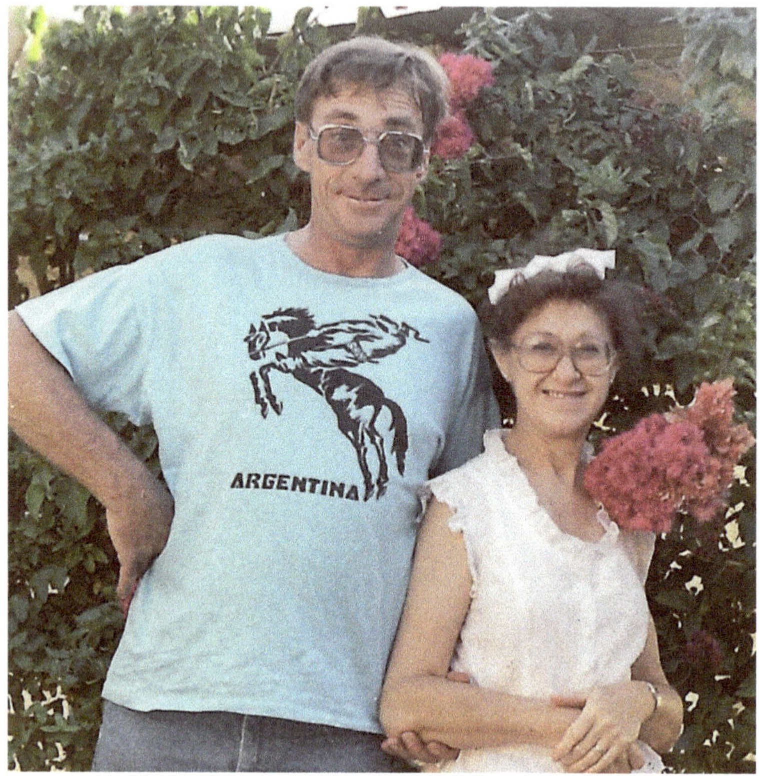

Visiting Stephen

As I lay in bed in Houston reminiscing about this final encounter, I felt her spirit near me, as if she had come to say goodbye to me from all those many miles away in Perth, Western Australia.

Ray and I decided to abandon our water sports interests and relegated ownership to our original mentor and investors. I would go home to Australia, as I expected a small inheritance from my mother's estate, while Ray would remain in Houston till our house was sold and then follow me home. Our little family would be reunited at last.

With a heavy heart, I started to prepare to leave the USA for the last time; however, I was looking forward to being with Stephen again and to help him with whatever he needed, saving me from the grief of losing my mother.

After sad farewells to my dear friends, Syble and her family, Shirley and her family and my beloved cat Oscar and dog Mandy, Ray drove me to Houston airport to catch my flight back home. Ray and I parted heartbroken again, and repeating history, I cried all the way back to Australia on my own.

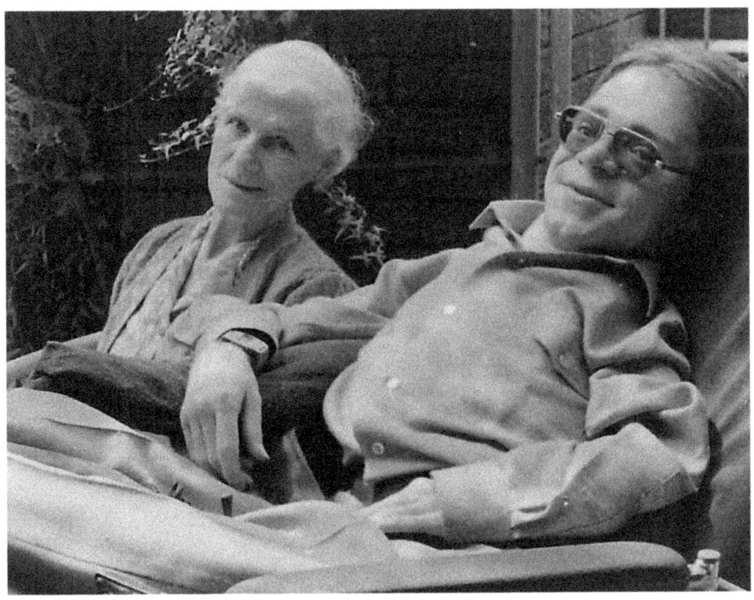

My mother with Stephen

PART 5: THE LATER YEARS

19

Back in Australia

I stayed with Ray's mother initially, before moving to Aunt Peg's place to be closer to Stephen. It felt so good to be close to my dear boy again.

I then set about looking for a job, having decided to look for one in a law firm. I applied for a word processing position that would train applicants, and went for an interview at a leading law firm in Perth. During my interview, however, the personnel manager started to gather her papers and seemed as if she was disinterested in hiring me. Since I was broke and desperately needed a job, I fell onto my knees and pounded her desk saying, "You have got to give me this job, please!"

She looked at me somewhat startled, then said, "Well, tell you what," and handed me a typewritten page. "Take this and type this exactly and bring it back when you have finished."

I typed as fast as I could with no errors and handed the page back to her. She was pleasantly surprised at my speed and accuracy and said I could start part-time from 1:30 PM the next week. With tears burning my eyes, I thanked her profusely and hurried home, feeling elated but nervous about what was in store for me.

In a couple of months – and helped with my mother's bequest – I had saved enough for a down payment on a small two-bedroom villa. Now I could have Stephen come stay weekends with me.

I had obtained a beautiful orange female tabby kitten through one of my workmates. Whenever Stephen arrived, the kitten would excitedly rush up to greet him, jumping up onto him and literally putting her two paws around his neck in a hug, purring all the while. We named her Buffy. She was a sweetheart who would snuggle contentedly in Stephen's lap all day. Unfortunately, Buffy succumbed to poison bait laid by someone who hated cats. I searched for days for her until a neighbour told me what had happened. Our hearts were broken. Buffy was just three years old when we lost her.

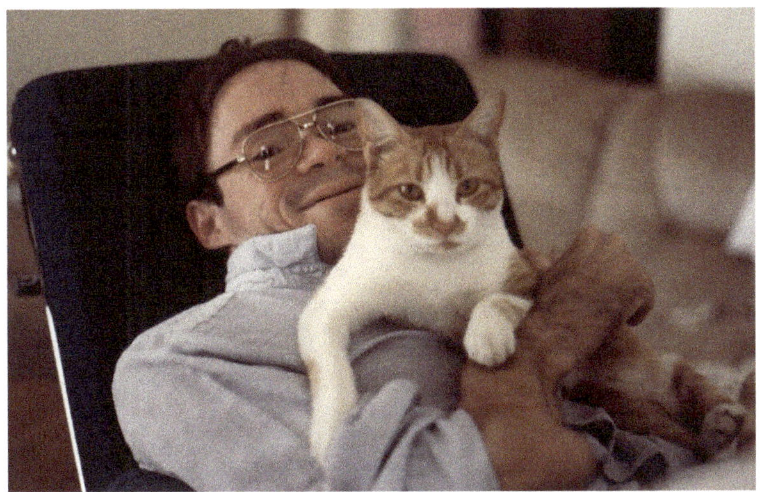

Stephen and Buffy

It took several months for our house in Houston, Texas, to be sold as the market was still depressed, but eventually Ray sold it for marginally less than what we had paid. He made a final trip to Nassau, Bahamas, collected $5,000 and the next day caught a plane from Miami to Perth, thus ending another disastrous episode in our tumultuous lives.

Ray found it difficult to break into the mining industry in Australia, and there was little or no manufacturing work available to match his skills. Some months later, he managed to find work on a small mine and was successful in implementing changes that increased its production and profitability. From then on, life took a turn for the better. With steady wages coming in, we soon paid off the debts that Ray had accumulated in America and started saving in earnest.

The next phase of Stephen's life was happier. He met more people who had a huge influence on him, and they in turn were inspired by his courage and many talents. He was happy that we were all together again.

Stephen became involved with the Project Coordinator, Philippa 'Pip' Daly Smith, who was in charge of the OT Department at his residence. Pip had developed a dedicated team of staff and volunteers to assist in the Department. This included the co-op where residents were encouraged to cultivate their interests and skills and, in many cases, to earn income.

An innovative co-op project that was initiated and developed with Stephen's input was the designing of electronic switches and connections that a person with a disability could easily use. This project was called the Switch-on Project. These special electronic devices enabled people with disabilities to use computers, communication aids or electronic toys, making electronics accessible to them for the first time and broadening their interests.

Stephen played a key role in making these adapted switches and enjoyed using his technological skills to both build the switches and to show other people how to use them. He was especially delighted when people with restricted movement purchased them and could use them to turn things on or off – something they previously had lacked the ability to do.

Pip enjoyed Stephen's passion for life, his talent for conversations, his unique sense of humour and wry observations about life, and his love of music. She told me his technological skills shone through despite his limited physical abilities. At this time, there were lots of new activities being introduced by Pip and her team of enthusiastic and devoted staff and volunteers. Stephen was keen to suggest new ideas and activities and happily participated in whatever way he could. His focus, of course, was technology and music.

A key aim of Pip's work was to create a homely environment for the mostly young male residents, which was a challenge since some had high support needs. Pip wanted to broaden their social life with parties, quiz nights, concerts and the introduction of computers.

One unforgettable night, Stephen went with a group of other residents, staff and volunteers from the facility to see the super star, Rod Stewart. To enable the group to see better, they were placed behind the metal rail barricade right near the stage. Everyone was enjoying the concert when Rod Stewart noticed the wheelchair-bound group and danced up close to sing to them. All at once the audience, totally oblivious of the people in wheelchairs sitting in front of them, rushed up to try to touch Rod, clambering over the vulnerable group.

Staff and volunteers, including Pip, immediately jumped up to link arms behind those in wheelchairs, trying with all their strength to hold back the audience as security staff rushed to their aid. Rod quickly grasped the danger of the situation himself and ran to the opposite side of the stage as the strong security staff lifted Stephen in his heavy wheelchair up and over to the other side of the rail barricade to safety. As a bonus, Stephen had the best seat in the house.

Changes were later made for future concerts by building a special viewing platform for wheelchair users where they could enjoy events safely.

The following report by Pip notes all the activities Stephen enjoyed:

OCCUPATIONAL THERAPY REPORT

December, 1985.

NAME: Steven Simpson

PERSONAL SKILLS AQUISITION PROGRAM:

Each person has an individual programme that is jointly decided by the person concerned and Occupational Therapy Staff.
This programme has specific goals that aim to help each individual develop to their full physical, social, emotional and intellectual potential. The programme is reviewed three times per year and runs to coincide with the school year.
Each person has a specific minimum number of hours that they ~~contract to do, usually 20 hours or more per week. (If they~~ do in excess of 20 hours they are elegible to apply for incentive and mobility allowances from the department of Social Security).

OT ACTIVITIES: The activities marked with an * are those that were included in Steven's OT programme this year.

WORK (Co-op Activities).

*Woodwork	Sewing Circle	Copperwire
*Dismantling	Stamps	Gardening Group
*Computer	Pay sheets	

Other activities specially negotiated.

SELF IMPROVEMENT AND OTHER ACTIVITIES.

*Jewellery making	Folk weaving	Weaving
Sewing	Mosaics	Gardening
Photography	Jigsaws	Woodburning
Art	Pottery	*Computers
China painting	*Cooking	Woodwork
Health and Beauty	Leatherwork	Typing
*Communication group	Brainbox	Video group
Independence group	*Quiz	*Shopping
Soccer	*Tech courses	News and views group

COMMENTS: (personal goals, special achievements, home modifications and aids etc).

1985 has been a year of excellent progress for Steven Simpson. He, during the year, has sorted out where he is going and what his priorities are. He has developed new interests and the ability to "follow through". This has been great to see and Steven is becoming more + more involved with various activities.
He has a great deal of creative ability and enjoys using the Macintosh computer in a most creative way.
He is a most valued member of the communication group and we look forward to see how Steven will further develop in 1986. Congratulations Steve!
You are a pleasure to have in O.T. (even filling in time sheets!!)

Philippa Daly Smith
(Occupational Therapist
In Charge).

Debbie Falck
(Occupational Therapist)

[illegible]

Despite his frail bones, Stephen longed to live a normal life. Fortunately, the nursing home encouraged residents to participate in 'normal' activities such as picnics and bus trips. These concepts may sound simple in nature; however, it took many volunteers to make the ideas eventuate. Volunteers are angels; they are the unsung heroes in any establishment.

The home where Stephen lived had a family-like organizational culture where volunteers and staff (who were often assisted by members of their own families) joined forces to take clients out and about or to throw an impromptu party. The volunteers were many and varied. They came with big hearts and the best of intentions, ceaselessly assisting residents like Stephen to achieve their rights to normality and unassumingly supporting them to reach their goals. Volunteers were highly valued and made life-changing contributions to residents' happiness. Their willingness to freely give and have fun lightened everyone's burdens.

Stephen's other great love was his Macintosh computer. John Curry, a retired World War II pilot who had flown missions on the Lancaster Bomber, volunteered many hours of his time helping Stephen learn about his computer. John was always there to help Stephen, thanks to which Stephen became a whiz on the system. These computers created huge benefits for people with disabilities, replacing boredom with a whole new world of opportunities while also developing creative and intellectual talents.

Another pleasurable activity for Stephen was the weekly cooking class run by Lois Mettam, a trained nurse and volunteer. She gave cooking lessons to a small group with disabilities including Stephen every week. Stephen had first met Lois during his time in Australia in 1974 and was much delighted to have her around the home still. Lois, an exceptionally beautiful soul, dedicated her life in helping her little group do food shopping to a budget, plan menus and supervise as they prepared and cooked meals.

Even after three hip replacements and being on crutches, through sheer love above and beyond, Lois would provide Christmas dinners for her group in her own home. She never forgot Stephen at Christmas, and for years marked his birthday by visiting him with beautiful handmade gifts and a homemade sponge cake.

Lois was presented with a plaque in 2006 for her life's service as a volunteer.

One day, Stephen's good friend Ric of the Aeolian Harp venture decided to cook a chocolate cake for everyone to enjoy for morning tea. These days, you would need about 20 different OHS (Occupational Health and Safety) certificates to gain access to the kitchen. Proud of himself, he placed the cake in the oven and eagerly waited for it to cook. Gradually, an odoriferous cloud of garlic filled the air. He had not realised that some of the residents had made garlic butter that same day and that's what he had used in the chocolate cake. Nobody was game enough to eat it, so he became the sole recipient of a large, garlic-flavoured chocolate cake amidst peals of laughter all around.

Stephen became friends with many of the personal carers assigned to him, resulting in several lasting friendships. Stephen thrived on conversations on every subject, from the real to the ridiculous. Much time was spent having fun lampooning the serious.

One such friend was Michael, a talented bass musician. Naturally, Stephen felt a strong kinship for him, given Michael's musical ability. They often played music together, with Michael on bass and Stephen on keyboard. Whenever Michael came to work, the first thing he would do was visit Stephen's room.

One particular day, Michael was stricken with grief. He had just heard the news of one of his best friends, with whom he had played much live music, having committed suicide. His friend's mother had nothing left of her son's music and was consequently even more heartbroken.

Michael had given Stephen a tape recording of him and his late friend playing together, and Stephen thought it would make a nice keepsake for the grieving mother. Stephen re-mixed it all with what is now considered primitive recording equipment. (This was prior to the digital age and programs like Garage Band.) He split it into individual tracks and adjusted sound levels. He then remastered the tape onto a chrome cassette with adjustments to the voice and mandolin tracks. It was labour-intensive work that took Stephen many hours and a lot of energy to complete.

Stephen used his gift of music to give the poor boy's grieving mother a lasting gift. Imagine the mother, who had long lost her husband and now lost both sons – one to suicide and one to a heart attack – receiving as a gift this music that her youngest son had made. She was 'thrilled to pieces' with the recording and thanked Stephen profusely for this memento to remember her son in happier times.

Romesh and Errol were two young architect students working as orderlies to pay for their university tuition. They provided not only good physical care but intellectual stimulation too. They had a positive effect on Stephen's remaining life, which was happy but too short. Romesh and Errol both went on to become senior lecturers in Architecture.

One of the happiest times for Stephen was at shower time. The bathroom had good acoustics, so Stephen was always laughing and singing at the top of his lungs with his good mate Romesh. Their favourite song to sing was by Gilbert and Sullivan: 'He is an Englishman!' from the comic opera H.M.S. Pinafore. They enjoyed singing the funny lyrics in operatic voices.

(Stephen sings)
He is an Englishman,
He is an Englishman,
For he, himself has said it,
And it's greatly to his credit,
That he is an Englishman!

(Romesh and Stephen sing)
He is an Englishman!

(Stephen sings)
For he might have been a Roosian,
A French, or Turk, or Proosian,
Or perhaps Itali-an

(Stephen and Romesh sing)
Or perhaps Itali-an!
But in spite of all temptations,
To belong to other nations,
He remains an Englishman!

In a letter Stephen wrote to me in February 1983, he illustrated their playfulness:

"Romesh is still great fun, keeps us laughing, always very witty, so witty it's not funny. Always does untold amount of work for everyone around here, including me. Plays cricket with the kids, takes people to movies, lets me have his autograph and take pictures of him. He asks me if I want a shower and I ask him if he wants one?"

In later years, every time before a major operation, Stephen would turn to Romesh for emotional support. Romesh responded happily.

Errol, a talented guitar player, generously shared his gift of music with the residents. He went on to make records and perform extensively around Australia. Interestingly, Errol has also composed music for orthopaedic surgery videos.

Errol said to me years later, "It was disabled people like Stephen who inspired me to make as much music as I could because I CAN – if

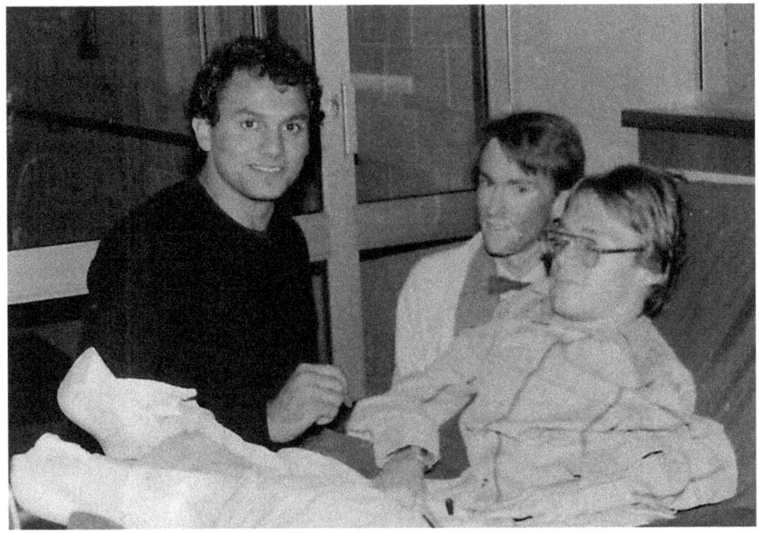

Romesh, Errol and Stephen

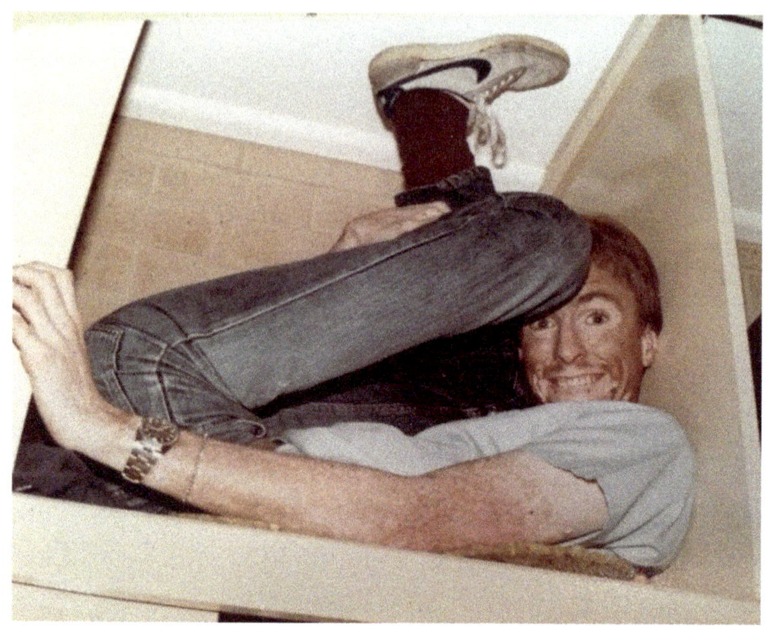

Errol's antics were always good for a laugh

that makes sense – and they would if they could. You can quote me on that if you like."

After showers were done, it was fun time. Errol would entertain residents with his mischievous antics, while Romesh and Stephen, with their love for English humour, would banter back and forth one-liners by Peter Cook and Dudley Moore, and from Monty Python skits. They had great appreciation for each other's sense of humour.

Here is Errol's story in his own words:

<u>The adventures of Stephen, Errol and various other 'silly' carers</u>

It was so long ago when I started working part time as a carer. I was studying architecture at university. The Matron found us architects not to be without intelligence, able to work unsupervised and not afraid of hard work. Her son was a carer and studying architecture himself. Soon the place was full of architecture students working as part-time carers.

Whilst not explicit in the job description, it seemed that an unwritten statement existed which said, 'all part-time carers shall, at all times, undertake their duties with due care and diligence. They shall also be quite silly whenever possible.' This was something I felt more ready to accept, as did many others on the team. Jokes aside, it was clear that our task was to put a smile on as many faces as possible in the short time we were there.

On Sunday we worked under the keen eye, steel temperament and iron will of the head nurse, who also possessed a magnificent heart of gold. Another feature of the day was Mrs Holly, the wonder cook, who turned on a fabulous roast lamb of which I was given a magnificent serve. I had cleaned her range exhaust without being asked. It was a very greasy and grizzly task most of the orderlies avoided. We had had a lecture that week at university on the dangers of commercial kitchens, especially the risk of fire from dirty, greasy exhaust grills. I had mentioned this to Mrs Holly and asked if she would like me to clean them for her. More fool me.

Many other things happened on a Sunday. The place turned into Monty Python, then Peter Cooke and Dudley Moore [well, Derek and Clive really]. There was also a guitar floating around that no one seemed to own, which I used to play if no pressing task required my attention. A lot of the kids were not familiar with having a live performer a metre from them. There was always time for a tune, and Lord knows I needed the practice. They were certainly not prepared for the sights of carers 'silly walking' down the corridors singing bizarre songs from the Monty Python catalogue, and lots worse.

The residents always seemed happy to see us. I think we were a fresh face at the end of what may have been a dull week for some. They knew we were on their side and also knew we were glad to see them. We seemed to develop a sense of humour that only existed at that place on those days.

There were some days when the kids were displaying 'cabin fever' symptoms. On such occasions, I often bundled up as many kids as possible into the little bus and took them for a drive to an interesting place like the docks when the ships were moored. Many songs were sung as we drove. The kids were good as gold when the boredom had ceased. Their residence returned to the pleasant [quiet] place it could be, and I got paid for looking at buildings I wanted to see, and the kids loved it.

Music was a large part of the lives of many of the residents. Some aspired to musicianship; Stephen was always keen to play music, especially Beatles songs. Those BLOODY Beatles songs. It was early days in my playing, and most of the subtleties in Beatles songs were a little beyond me. This didn't stop Stephen. He kept belting out the melody while I clumsily attempted the many chords flying by on the sheet music. I am pretty happy that no copies of the 'Sunday tunes sessions' exist. Our Sunday music sessions were less than sparkling, but Stephen enjoyed the chance to be a musician for even a short while. Oddly enough, we did not develop regular audiences. I am pretty sure John Lennon was turning in his grave – apologies, John.

I feel that Stephen, and others, were an inspiration for me to pursue music. There was so much he would have done if his body had not let him down. I had no such excuse, so what was stopping me?

I ended up making records, performing and doing all sorts of oddball things with music. Music has taken me all around the world. Who else do you know who survived a gig full of 200 very scary bikies, then made music for orthopaedic surgery videos? I have made 16 albums of my original guitar music. Both my PhD and Masters were about music, sound and architecture. I have had cancer since 2012, and I have used music as a healing force. The results so far have been quite remarkable, even though I can offer no scientific evidence to support that statement.

What did I learn? I learned about caring for people and how to not be afraid to touch people; any bodily waste in the bathroom presents no challenge for this little fella. This [slightly] prepared me for the early days of fatherhood. I learned that disabled people appreciate your help but despise your sympathy, which is no use to them at all. I learned that disabled people are not freaks, and many of them have done quite a lot with seemingly little. I often feel the need to say to folks addressing a disabled person: "The person you are speaking to is disabled, not DEAF!"

When I see a person in a wheelchair struggling to load their groceries into their car, I move into 'orderly mode' without thinking and help them get it all safely on board. When I see someone wounded, I have no difficulty addressing the wound and the person. Variations

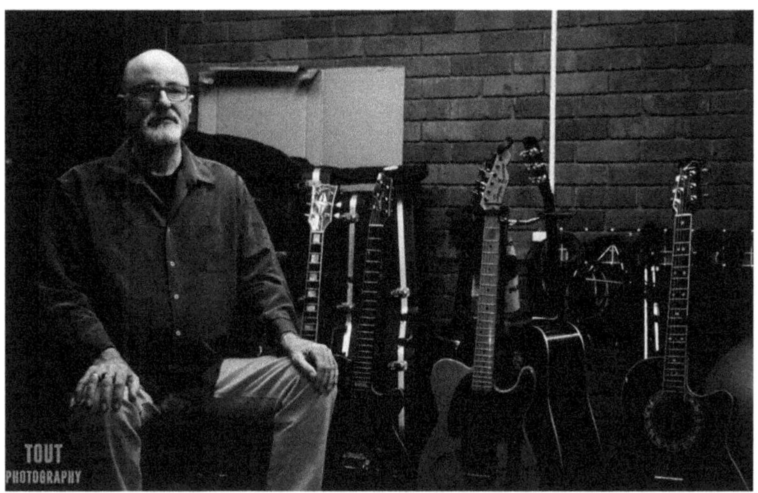

photo of Errol Tout taken by Sam Tout

of this scenario happen all the time. I also learned to not feel sorry for myself, no matter the situation. This unquestionably has been useful in the treatment of my cancer.

I also learned about death, as it was commonplace there. I don't fear it and sometimes see it as a positive release for those suffering unbearably.

20

The Best Band

Although Ray's work was temporary in nature, his skills were always in demand and his remuneration increased with every position, so much so that we soon bought a block of land in a new subdivision. Ray and Stephen set about designing a house, with large rooms and wheelchair accessibility throughout. Ray and I moved into our new house in 1990.

Stephen's nursing home, like any establishment, was a place of both light and shadows. There was a group of staff and patients who often partied together. It was like a big family, and as in any family, there were members who got on well with each other and others who did not. Indeed, there were some truly bright lights to be grateful for.

Stephen was delighted to see his old friend Ric, the wheelchair technician who had built the carrier for him when we travelled back to America, still working in the workshop. He developed a great relationship with him. They spent many hours of fun together listening to the Beatles and The Fabulous Poodles.

Due to Stephen's love of stringed instruments and his fascination with sound, Stephen requested Ric to build an Aeolian harp, and he good-naturedly agreed. Now a days, people would say that's not in their job description, but Ric only said, "I have had to make some funny things in my time, but this is one of the funniest."

The Aeolian or wind harp is named after the Greek God, Aeolus. It is a harp that is literally played by the wind. It can range in size from small trinkets to large structures and makes eerie siren-like sounds when a strong wind is blowing. Ric extended some strings, so they stretched taut between two posts situated in a wind passage. He tried to alternate with long and short strings for different pitches to sound beautiful and haunting. Stephen would sit in his wheelchair giving instructions.

Ric tried valiantly to get the harp to work but alas, it was a dismal failure. All of us laughed over it.

Staff and patients were allowed to drink and smoke together. Patients in their wheelchairs, including Stephen, 'danced' at parties as joyously as any able-bodied persons. Long-term employees were not uncommon at the facility; it was rewarding to work closely with the residents.

The CEO would often take a break from his busy day to hand-deliver mail to every patient. If people questioned the merit of him doing a mailman's mundane duty, perhaps they did not understand that it was, in fact, an incredibly smart move. It made him very approachable, and he knew every employee and every patient by name.

"Morning, Stephen! Here is a letter for you," he would announce as he strode briskly into his room. It gave him a natural opening to then ask, "How are you?" He was in charge, but still in touch with everyone. The management was open to ideas that would benefit residents, whose welfare and happiness came first.

Music for Stephen was the essence of life itself and played a huge role in giving meaning to his existence. The Beatles music remained the greatest love of his whole life. He expanded his knowledge and taught himself techniques to record with sound perfectly onto cassette tapes. He had the gift to play music by ear on his keyboard using only his right hand. He especially loved electronic music composers such as Jean Michel Jarre, Vangelis and Isao Tomita playing on synthesizers.

Stephen listened to music with a very discerning ear, able to hear small details that others would miss. One day, while playing a Beatles song for me, he repeatedly pointed out the sound where Ringo, their drummer, dropped his drumstick to the floor. I listened intently over and over as he patiently pointed out the precise second the drumstick dropped, but try as I might I could not pick up this intricate sound.

Valued support for Stephen came from Jane Anne. She initially worked as an Occupational Therapy Assistant in a little open office in the Day Centre. From here she could see residents as they came to and from the Matron's office. Because the office was adjacent to the open area, people would often stop and talk with her. There was a steady stream of visitors in wheelchairs. Jane Anne was not directly involved in participating as a care provider, but she was the ideal sounding board for the residents. She listened.

Stephen became a daily visitor to her office. She recognised Stephen as being intelligent and therefore they had an adult-level connection. Stephen found in her a safe and secure place to share his frustrations. Jane Anne observed Stephen's difficulties in dealing with his life and pain. She understood with her heart and soul where Stephen was coming from. In turn, Stephen taught her a lot about life in general.

Stephen was a natural teacher. He had the capacity to help people help him. He meticulously taught them how to handle him with care without resorting to complaints or orders. He never accepted the standard of second-best or near-enough being good enough. He liked things to be just right. He was sure the staff did not know the depth of his pain and therefore they could not understand it.

Jane Anne also mentioned Stephen taught her other key lessons: the importance of respect for all people and the value of kindness. Although Stephen was permanently beset with pain, he always had a twinkle in his eye and a lot of courage in his heart. She added that he had taught her about humility and humanity, what life is like for the disabled residents, and how easy it is to be kind. Certainly, we all have jobs to do, but is injecting kindness and humour into our interactions with others really that hard? There is no financial outlay required, just a soft heart.

Three exceptional musicians, Linda Blyth, Sue Hadley and Roger Montgomery, all employees of the nursing home, had an idea to start up a band with whoever was interested. Of course, Stephen was highly motivated to participate.

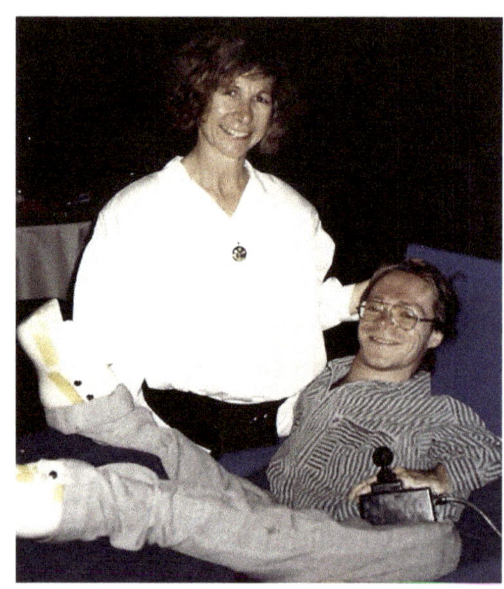
Jane Anne and Stephen

Linda was a member of Occupational Therapy (OT) staff and a clarinettist and singer. Sue Hadley was a Registered Music Therapist and cellist and singer. Roger Montgomery is a well-known folk guitarist, singer, songwriter and poet. In the 1980s and '90s, he was leader of the Mucky Duck Bush Band as well as a care assistant. Sue went on to get a Masters in Music Therapy in America and became a Professor of Music Therapy. Linda went on to become a Registered Music Therapist and OT and works in Bunbury, Western Australia. Roger still does the National Folk Circuit.

Altogether, these artists and residents pulled together to form The Travelling Wheelchairies band, which was loosely modelled around a popular British American supergroup of that time: The Traveling Wilburys, with lead singer Tom Petty performing bass and vocals. Sadly, Tom Petty died on October 2, 2017, at age 66. Other members in this diverse singer-songwriter super group were: Bob Dylan, guitar; Jeff Lynne, guitar; Jim Keltner, drums; Roy Orbison, guitar and vocals (died December 6, 1988 at age 52); and former Beatle George Harrison, guitar and vocals (died November 29, 2001, at age 58).

It was a happy time for Stephen. Being with the music group was instrumental in relieving stress for him, saving him from depression and lessening his pain. He always focused on keyboards, synthesisers

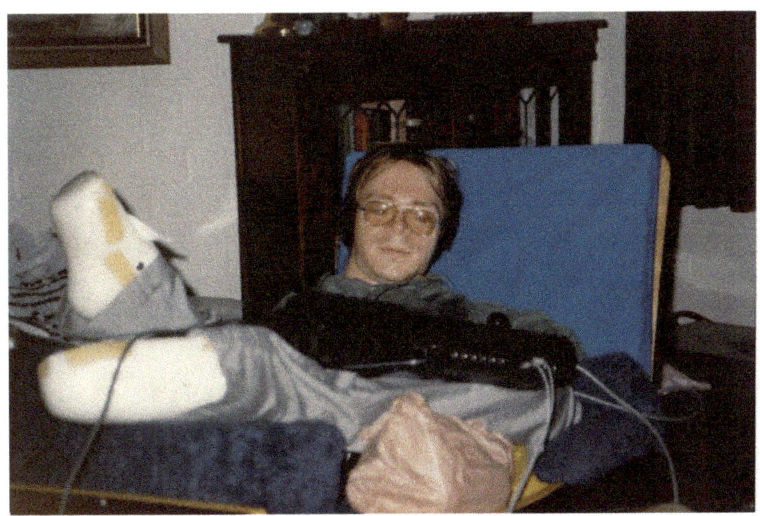

Stephen working with music, mixing for sound recording

and guitars. He loved to mix music; he could be creative, becoming lost in the beauty of music. It was an outlet for expressing the feelings that his physical condition precluded him from achieving in any other manner.

Linda had a percussionist friend who kindly donated an old drum kit, whose separate parts could be played by different individuals depending on their physical ability. Many musical instruments were donated from various sources including a local music shop.

The members in the band with Stephen had various disabilities ranging from:

- *Duchenne Muscular Dystrophy,* a genetic disorder characterised by progressive muscle degeneration and weakness.
- *Friedreich's Ataxia,* a disease that causes progressive damage to the nervous system resulting in poor coordination and a number of neurological disorders.
- *Spina bifida,* a malformation of the spine where the spine does not completely close, exposing the spinal cord. Most sufferers have some degree of weakness or paralysis in their lower limbs.
- *Thalidomide defects:* Thalidomide was given to pregnant women in the 1950s and 1960s to treat morning sickness but was removed from sale in 1961 after it was linked to birth defects. Babies were born with deformities including the absence of arms and legs.

Each band member played an instrument that was best suited to their ability. None were impaired cognitively. People often assume physical impairment coincides with intellectual impairment, or that a disabled person is deaf and has to be shouted at; people talk over them and not to them. The disabled person can pick this up immediately.

Being in the band was not only helpful for Stephen, but it also benefited all the members. With their disabilities and special needs, they had a right to a normal non-judgemental individual existence which was enabled by the support of their team leaders.

The group met weekly, cementing friendships through music. They shared with each other their favourite songs. There were lots of laughter as they wrote compositions to known melodies. This special time gave a space for band members to broaden their outlook and take turns really listening to one another. It helped them to think for themselves, to express their own likes and dislikes and to grow in directions beyond institutionalisation and dependency. Of course, Stephen won everyone over to appreciate the Beatles music that he always played.

The Travelling Wheelchairies went on to develop a wide repertoire of music. Songs they played ranged from 'Am I Ever Going to See your Face Again' by the Angels, to 'Beach Shack' and 'Don't Be Cruel' by Elvis, to 'You Shook me All Night Long' by AC/DC. Playing such a wide range of music broadened Stephen's musical appreciation skills.

They decided as a group to put on a show to showcase their skills and talents. It was a wonderful opportunity for the band members to develop teamwork skills as they had to learn to not only work together, but to plan, set up and host the show as well as to play music for the show. The high quality of the music produced was enjoyed by all who attended, and it was made more special by the fact that the band members overcame significant physical challenges to make the music. I was beaming with pride and my heart bursting with joy to see Stephen playing in his band after all his hard work.

The care home newsletter printed:

> *The debut performance by The Travelling Wheelchairies, co-led by Susan Hadley and Roger Montgomery, provided an opportunity for these residents to exhibit the skills they have developed since the band's inception six months ago. Proud parents and friends watched, and nerves were put to the test as the band played on.*
>
> *Steven Simpson, one of the organisers and a member of the band said:*
>
> *"There were a lot of kids sitting in the front row. Roger stopped the band and got the audience involved and motivated to join in. It was good fun. It was more fun playing to an audience that joined in, shouting and screaming together. It took the pressure off us."*

It did not matter if the music was commercially made or if it came from the Travelling Wheelchairies, all music brought Stephen much joy.

Stephen's physical condition, unfortunately, continued to decline, particularly the state of his legs. The bones had shrunk to the same diameter as a pencil and just the force of gravity could break them. Because Stephen's legs were so fragile and his knees did not bend, much time had to be invested in the careful handling of his legs to prevent stress fractures.

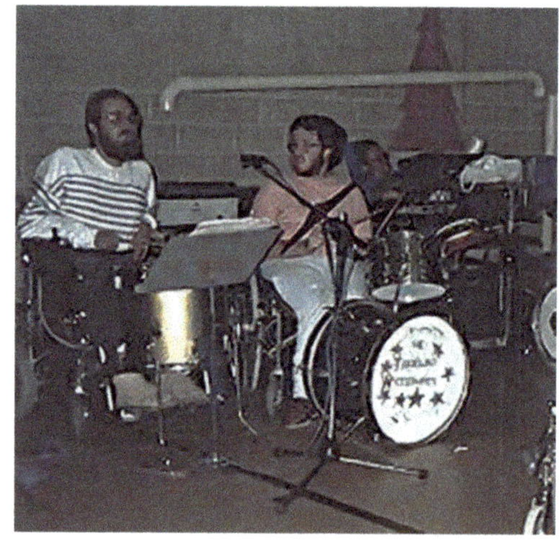

Stephen in the background with two of his mates, Lance and Michael

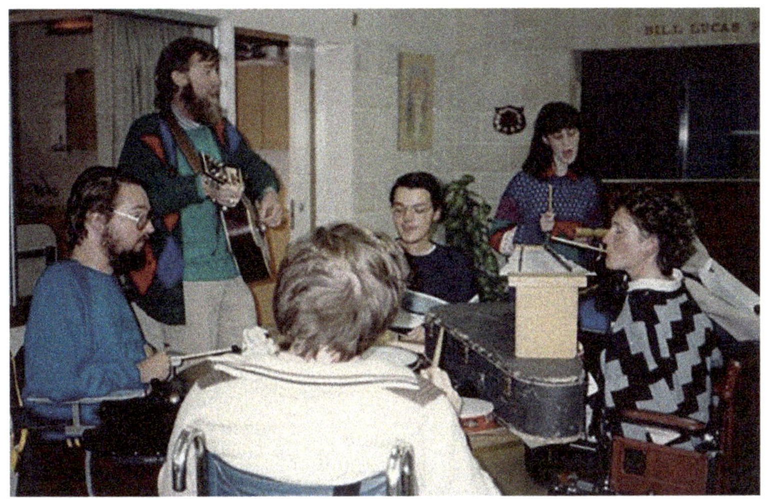

Band members Lance, Roger, Barney, Sue, Monica and Michael (back to camera)

One day, Stephen's doctor suggested, "You'd be better off without those legs. Have you considered amputation?"

When Stephen told me of this shocking suggestion, I felt sick and could not sleep for three weeks thinking about this bizarre proposition. It struck fear and shock in our hearts. Stephen was visibly upset with this idea and was struggling to put on a brave face despite his depression. So we rejected the idea.

It was only three years later, when I realised one day what he had to tolerate just to get ready for his shower, that amputation began to make a great deal of sense. Thereafter, thoughts about the amputation started to come into my mind more frequently.

By then his legs had frequent stress fractures. The pain involved in lifting his legs in and out of the braces prior to showering, then drying them and placing them carefully back into his braces, was crushing to watch. Due to their inherent weakness, his legs were continuously encased in plastic splints for support and were now frozen directly in front of him. Due to this inflexibility, Stephen required an extension to his wheelchair. This made negotiation through doorways challenging. It was difficult to get close to reach anything, and transportation in general more cumbersome. His legs were the source of constant pain, requiring ever stronger analgesics to mitigate his suffering.

While observing his daily care, I began writing a list of why Stephen would be better off without his painful legs. This included less physical discomfort, more ease of bathing, less stress getting his pants on, ability to engage in outings with less fuss and therefore less pain. Altogether, I came up with 12 reasons why Stephen should have this radical surgery.

One day, I showed my list to Stephen and he agreed with my reasons. Unknown to me, he had been making notes himself about his own fears, which clearly showed how he was building up his courage to have the operation. He pondered about having his legs off. 'Because they were useless' was not a good enough reason. He wondered how he would deal with life after the operation. Would he still lie in bed as much in a day? Would he be able to sit up easily and for how long? Would being without legs be a strain to his lower back?

Stephen asked several friends if they thought he should have the operation, but not everyone understood his plight and he was in unknown territory trying to make this decision. One friend responded jokingly, "Lying around in bed all day sounds like a good idea to me, but you won't know what reasons you had for keeping your legs until you take them away."

His doctor explained that cutting a limb may sometimes cause pain to move up to a higher place in the body. This was something to contemplate. Stephen also wondered if he would experience ongoing phantom limb pain. His biggest fear was about fractures to other parts of his body during the operation. He was anxious about being lifted while he was unconscious; the dead weight of his body could cause fractures unless his body was fully supported.

Along came a new friend named John who had been the victim of a virus that had left him paralysed and deaf in 1989. After a year of physiotherapy, some movement had come back into his left arm and leg, and his hearing had returned. Stephen considered John a valuable asset to the facility, as he had had a normal upbringing and had not been institutionalised from birth like some of the other residents. John thought outside the paradigm, resulting in good conversations with Stephen.

With John came his girlfriend Adriana, and thoughts of amputation were put into the back of Stephen's mind.

21

Lost and Found

Adriana had been John's girlfriend for three years when he fell sick with the virus. When Stephen met them, their relationship was starting to spiral downward. John felt she only stayed in the relationship because he was waiting on an insurance payout for a previous car accident. Adriana wanted John's disability pension to be paid into her bank account, but John wisely declined. By early 1991, John separated from Adriana.

Knowing she could not manage financially on her own, she decided to become Stephen's girlfriend. Her plan was to get Stephen to live with her, sharing rent and living expenses. Subsequently, she would be his carer. She wanted Stephen to give her control of his disability pension, so she could be in full charge of the financial arrangements. That part of her plan didn't eventuate, which was lucky for Stephen.

They began to chat more and more. For a time, she continued to be friends with both John and Stephen. Stephen did not feel that she looked at him as disabled; he insisted she looked at him from her heart, or so he thought.

She visited Stephen three times per week, doing many kind things for him, and so Stephen fell in love with her. He thought the world of her. It was refreshing for Stephen to have a very pretty girlfriend, and it did much for his self-esteem. He would sit up for as long as he could even with so much pain, just to not appear so disabled.

Imagine sitting in a nursing home in a wheelchair, thinking your days are over and dealing with chronic pain daily, and then an attractive young woman walks in and announces she would like to be your girlfriend!

When we fall in love, the area of the brain responsible for judgement shuts down, and we are less likely to be critical or sceptical of the person we care about. With love, fear and negative emotions reduce, which can also make us feel euphorically happy. For Stephen, experiencing this love was a wonderful new feeling that gave him some release from his pain. Stephen thought he had found a safe harbour of emotional safety. He thought he had found a companion to help him navigate life's turbulent waters.

And so it was that Stephen fell deeply in love with her, not imagining it would all come crashing down and break his heart.

Around this time, I decided a dog and cat were needed for happiness and company. Aunt Peg told me of a friend whose dog had just had pups. I went to look at them and came back with the latest family addition. She was just a Heinz variety, but she became Stephen's most lovable companion. We named her Elly May Clampett after Elly May in the Beverly Hillbillies.

She knew instinctively how to be gentle by carefully walking around Stephen on his bed. Stephen would tie her leash to his electric wheelchair, and she would jog alongside him, never pulling too fast. She had a beautiful connection with him, and he would often speak to her in 'dog speak' that only she could understand.

Soon after, I obtained a beautiful tabby kitten. I named her Barbara Ann after the Beach Boys song. Then came a calico cat named Syble Jean. Our family was now complete, and our pets provided company and a distraction for Steve's ever-present pain.

While reading the newspaper one morning, I came across an article about a doctor who treated people with OI. I immediately wrote him a letter discussing Stephen's recommended amputation. Consequently, a visit was arranged and when the doctor saw Stephen, it was agreed he would be better off without his painful legs. Stephen's quality of life had long been impaired by his atrophied legs.

Stephen continued to wrestle with this decision and consulted freely with Ray and I, as well as his carers, friends, surgeon and even his Pastor. Stephen's faith was deep and had sustained him through many trials. Eventually, he made the enormous decision to undergo the double amputation.

Naturally, Stephen was nervous and worried about his legs being amputated. We reassured him as much as we could over and over that everything would be better, explaining how he would be able to do so much more and endure less pain.

Stephen talked to his old friend Romesh about his fears and asked him to come to the hospital to see him on the day of his surgery. As it happened, Romesh had a relative who was a doctor, and by a stroke of luck, he would be assisting the surgeon in the operation. This good doctor sat with Stephen the day before the amputation. He listened carefully to Stephen's many fears about the surgery. Stephen explained if he were moved or lifted the wrong way during the surgery, it could cause a bone to snap. While he was awake, he would remain calm instructing his carers step by step how he was to be handled, but while he was asleep, he had no control over how he was handled.

Unlike an able-bodied person with an illness, Stephen would go into a hospital disabled and come out still disabled or in a worse condition due to further accidental injuries. On a few occasions, Stephen had been admitted to hospital for a broken bone, only to come out with more bones broken. How unfair is that?

The doctor reassured Stephen he would make sure all his instructions were duly followed when handling his unconscious body during surgery, to reduce the risk of fracture. This was a profound relief for Stephen that helped alleviate his many worries and made it able for him to trust the doctors.

Stephen, Ray and I were extremely anxious and nervous on the day of Stephen's operation. When we arrived at the hospital, we were informed that Stephen wanted his parents to prepare him for the procedure. The nurses were a big help as Ray and I got him ready. They brought us a tray filled with everything needed to prepare Stephen's legs for the surgery. We showered and towel dried him and then proceeded to shave his legs. I concentrated hard not to cut him, recalling all the times in the past when nurses had accidently cut his skin by holding the razor carelessly.

Stephen was agitated and kept talking about why the operation may not be the right thing to do. He thought of many strategies for postponing the operation. He clearly was using delaying tactics for his peace of mind. We repeatedly reminded him of the reasons why we had agreed he would be better off without his legs, even though I could fully feel his anxiety and panic myself. My heart was pounding with fear of the unknown and the frantic hope that we had made the right decision.

After giving detailed instruction to the surgical crew regarding how to lift and place him on the operating table and how to position his weak left arm, we walked beside him down the corridor to the operating room doors. I knew he was traumatised by seeing the lights above flashing by on the way to the theatre with fear of the unknown from so many operations, so many times before. Claire told me that Stephen told her he had had 47 surgeries in his life. The waiting surgical crew then took Stephen, and he disappeared from our sight into the operating theatre.

All his past surgeries had been traumatic, but none came close to the anxiety we experienced during this one.

After five or so hours of waiting for what was supposed to be a three-hour operation, a theatre nurse came to tell us that one leg had been amputated and everything was going well, but that the surgeon was having trouble disentangling some nerves behind his other knee; she assured us it would all be over soon.

After a total of nine hours, Stephen was wheeled into the recovery room and we were allowed to see him. His face was completely ashen, and he was connected to numerous tubes and machines with his stumps laid out on pillows. We were once again assured that he was doing well.

I fought back tears as he woke up. He gingerly moved his neck (to see if it worked okay), then lifted his right arm tentatively. It was all okay. We knew then he was going to be all right. Sheer joy replaced my tears. He was all in one piece with no broken bones. He had faced this operation so courageously. My stomach stopped turning and I began to feel relieved. It had been a long day.

We called Adriana and his nursing home and told them Stephen's operation was over and that he was doing fine. They sent him a card with everyone signing it, praising him for his courage.

After making sure Stephen was comfortable, we left feeling happy. The surgery had been a success, relieving all our fears. As we were

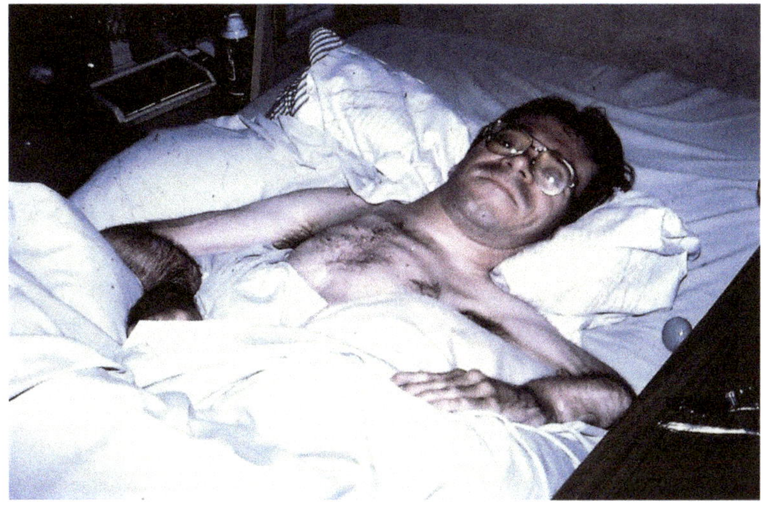

My poor boy in great pain after both legs were amputated below his knees

walking down the corridors, we were delighted to see Romesh coming towards us. We greeted him excitedly with the good news, feeling even happier that seeing Romesh would be the best treat in the world for Stephen.

Steve's friend John visited soon after. He made him laugh when the first thing he said was: "You're two feet shorter, short of two feet!" John's witty remark was remembered between them for a good laugh for many years thereafter.

When Stephen returned to the residence, the doctor had his wheelchair cut back for under his legs to make it easier for him to manoeuvre. All the nurses and his friends shouted and cheered Stephen. They made jokes saying they wanted their legs cut off too.

It was immediately noticed that his care requirements had significantly decreased. Less daily intervention was needed to prevent fractures of his tibias. Who would have thought an amputation meant freedom? Yet that was the most helpful operation he ever had.

Stephen purchased an engagement ring for Adriana to further cement their relationship. He then began planning to get a place for him and Adriana to live. He soon found that while it was not easy to get into a nursing home, getting out came with its own set of challenges.

He was interviewed by psychologists and occupational therapists to assess if he was suitable to leave their care. Stephen felt the reports were biased – based on the stresses of being in care and without the knowledge of how he would behave in a different environment. The reports took forever. One doctor did not return a letter to get the psychologist report started, and then it took another six weeks to get a reply. Stephen clung on to the hope that Adriana would be his carer.

Eventually, Adriana found a small apartment and Stephen finally moved to begin his new life. Initially it was all harmonious. Soon, though, standards of care started to disappear. Stephen was often left unable to reach for necessities. He was left alone for long periods of time without food or water or anything he needed. He even arranged to return to the nursing home for his daily shower.

Stephen called me one day, and I was shocked to hear them over the phone screaming at each other. Stephen was terribly upset and told me Adriana had been out all day, leaving him to fend for himself. I said, "You're coming home. I am coming to get you now."

And so his hopes for independence and a normal life were dashed.

Stephen was devastated but continued to love her for a long time. With our support and John's encouragement, and of course his music, he gradually came to see her true colours as a heartless opportunist. He would often say then that she would never realise how much he had loved her.

Somehow my soldier boy got through this calamity and later was able to laugh about it. John and Stephen would not use her name, and when speaking of her she was referred to as 'the unmentionable'. Although the breakup was very painful for him, he matured with wisdom for helping others.

Coming home with us to live and having new carers made Stephen much happier. He was able to choose his own carers and pay them with Government funding, giving him some independence and control.

A wonderful, gentle young lady named Kelly, who Stephen had met previously, was his carer for four valuable years, together with his old friend Lester and Claire, who was a student nurse. All of them shared rosters in supporting Stephen's care. These beautiful compassionate people all became dedicated friends, devoted to making Stephen's life the best it could be.

When each of our wonderful carers moved on, I would cry my heart out, but inevitably another would soon come into our lives. They were all Godsent, another example of good coming out of bad. Furthermore, I contemplated, if good comes out of bad, then how can anything be bad?

Another organisation was put into place to come each evening to help make Stephen comfortable for the night and placing everything within his reach. Each morning before I left for work, I would get Stephen ready for the first carer to arrive at 11 AM. As soon as I got to work, I would phone him to see if he was okay, and again at 11 AM to make sure the carer had arrived. It all worked well for a few years.

Then one day, we were informed that homes were being built for disabled people to live independently in the community, and a house was being built for Stephen too. This was a new phase in his life. We thought this move would be good for Stephen and give him more independence and control of his life. However, lurking round the corner was disaster lying in wait.

You see, in an institution it is normal to be disabled, but in the community, it is abnormal to be disabled.

In time, Stephen moved from our house to his new home with his carers Lester and Claire, and a new carer named Brad, who matched Stephen's witty humour. Brad stayed with Stephen for 11 years as his carer and remained his close friends for 17 years.

Stephen did not have a carer for night time, leaving him defenceless and vulnerable if someone broke in. So I would go over to Stephen's house with a cooked dinner and take our dog Elly May to stay the night, then make Stephen comfortable the next morning till the carer arrived before setting out to work.

What followed was one calamity after another. We lost Elly May when she was hit by a car. I took her to the vet, but she had to be put to sleep as her back had been broken. Needless to say, we both reached a new low. With a mixture of utter sadness and anger, I said to Stephen, "It is all too hard, Stevie, and I think it would be easier for the both of us if you just come back home, son."

Ray was working away most of the time in Fiji and only came home for a week every month. I was left alone to run two houses, manage Stephen's many needs, and juggle my own job at a busy law firm. Stephen coming home could cut my work and stress in half.

Brad put a notice in his church asking for a carer for Stephen. Linda, another great girl who was in training to be a nurse, answered. Linda helped me to pack Stevie's belongings and after a few trips between both our houses, we were home again. It was instant relief, and I was happy knowing I could make Stephen's life better now.

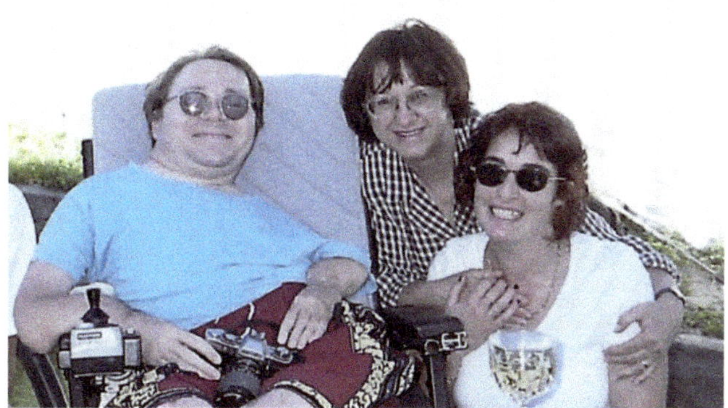

Stephen, me and Linda

22

Ob-La-Di, Ob-La-Da, Life Goes On

Barring Ray's frequent absence working on different gold mines, we were all together now. Our house was filled with a variety of music, from classical to the Beatles, played by Stephen.

Again, it was time for another dog. This time I brought home a Jack Russell puppy. We named her Lilly Little Legs. She was a wonderful companion to Stephen, always on his bed, and careful and gentle just like Elly May. Even though both dogs were acquired years apart, they both instinctively knew how to contain their boundless energy when spending time with Stephen. It was like they had a sixth sense about being careful to avoid hurting Stephen. Lilly Little Legs and Stephen had many great conversations again in 'dog speak' with Lilly listening intently to Stephen's every word.

Lilly was a great protector. One day while out the front of our house, she noted a man letting his three German Shepherds out of his car at the end of the street. Lilly at once took off at high speed towards the German Shepherds. The man saw Lilly coming towards them and quickly bundled the three dogs back into the car. Three German Shepherds and a man were afraid of Lilly Little Legs! What a laugh we had at Lilly's protectiveness!

I started line dancing, which introduced me to many new fun friends. We all would dance at various clubs several times a week. I had wonderful neighbours, a couple with five daughters. Each would sit with Stephen in turn when I was out dancing. I was worry free for an hour, knowing he was in good hands.

One night after dancing, I called my sitter and told her I was on my way home, so she left. I asked my friend Stella if she could go into my house with me just to see everything was all right as Ray was away working. I found I did not have a key to get in, so we proceeded to walk around the house looking for an open window. We came to Stephen's room and knocked on the window and told him through the glass that we were locked out. Of course, he could not do anything about the situation but called back with his quick wit, "Do you want a pillow?"

His comment gave us fits of laughter. We finally pulled off the flyscreen and were able to open the window and crawled through, still laughing hysterically at his remark.

We began to host themed dress-up parties for each of our birthday, anniversaries, Christmas – or any excuse for a party. Since Stephen was limited as to a social life, our friends contributed with social events at our house. These parties were great fun. All the carers would come, catering to Stephen's every little need.

At one party we had an Elvis impersonator as a surprise for Stephen's birthday. The music was so loud that the police came to our front door saying a neighbour had complained about the noise.

At another party, we had Sylvester and Tweety Bird balloons filled with helium floating among the guests. A door was left open, and Sylvester and Tweety inched their way towards the door. Once they were at the door, they suddenly swooped outside and quickly rose skyward.

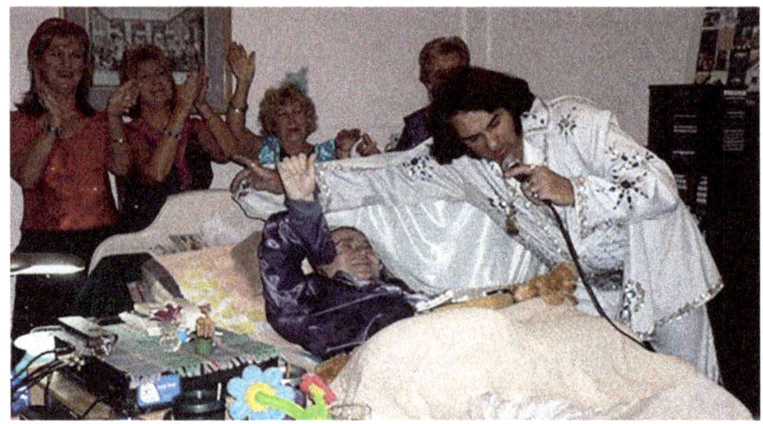

Steve and 'Elvis'

Everyone was jumping up trying to catch the feet of Sylvester and Tweety Bird, even as they were way out of reach and ascending fast. I didn't know whether to laugh or cry. Stephen was amazed watching the unfolding commotion, but a little disappointed as the balloons went higher and higher into the unknown.

We all laughed when we saw the news being reported later: "Sylvester and Tweety Bird were seen hovering over and around the city."

Ray and I were both working and earning good salaries. We paid off our house debt and went world travelling every year. We were grateful to Stephen's carers as they cared for Stephen, the house, the dog and two cats in our absence. They did a wonderful job and gave us peace of mind while we were away.

We travelled mostly by cruise ship. I was somewhat restricted on which activities I could undertake due to being unable to walk long distances. With Ray's help pulling me up mountains and steep stairs, sometimes even carrying me, I managed to see most places.

Before the days of the Internet and Skype, we telephoned Stephen every day from wherever we were, making sure he was going well. He

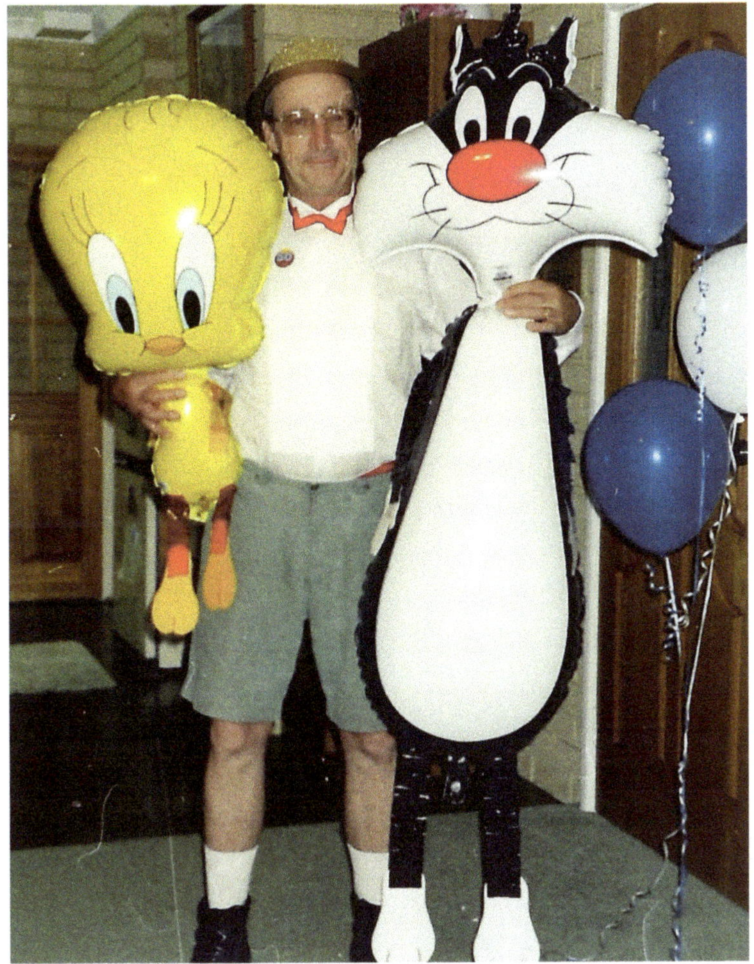

Ray with Sylvester and Tweety Bird

was thrilled listening to our adventures. Sometimes we were unable to connect from long distance or the operators were speaking every language you could think of except English. We would then rely on postcards to communicate.

Because Stephen was not able to come with us, we were determined to include him in seeing the world with us by phone calls and Skype. He would research little known facts about our locations. His

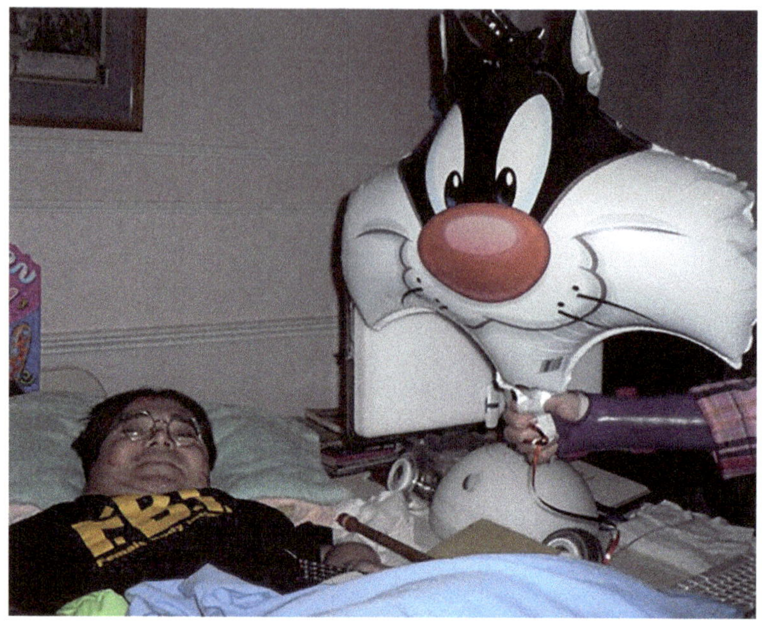

Steve, in his FBI shirt, and Sylvester

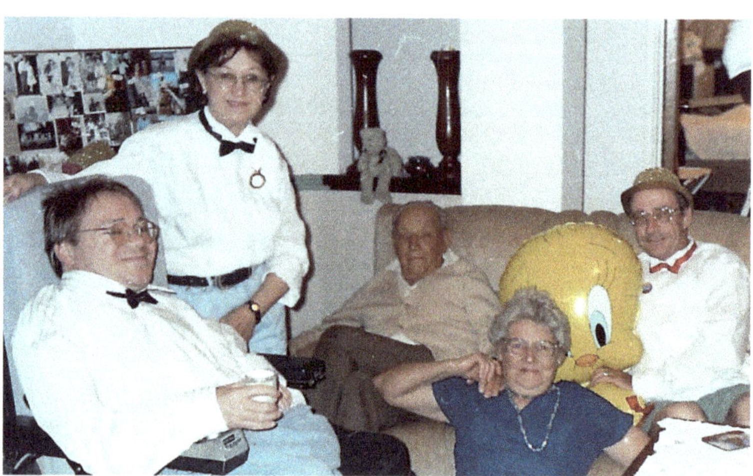

Stephen's 39th birthday party with us and Ray's dad and Alice, his second wife

knowledge of places around the world was enhanced even more. It was a distraction from his pain, keeping his mind stimulated. He would follow us everywhere through Google maps on his computer.

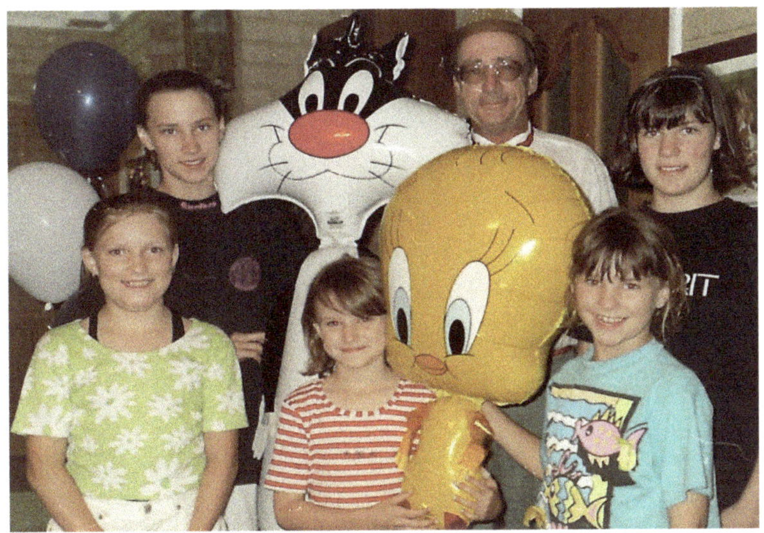

Ray with our neighbour's daughters

This gave Stephen great material for conversation with his carers who were always eagerly awaiting any news. Stephen's best friend Claire would frequently stay in our house while we were away to make sure all was well.

We traversed the globe to the far ends. Whilst on a ship in Panama, the Captain announced our loved ones could access a website to view the scenery captured by our ship's cameras as we were passing through the Panama Canal. Stephen told us he could see our ship and the beautiful vistas unfolding around us. We were delighted to share this experience with him.

Stephen continued to follow our travels on the internet to Spain, including to Madrid, Salamanca, Toledo, Barcelona, Valencia and Alhambra, onward to Venice, Dubrovnik and Split. Our ship sailed around the beautiful islands of Greece. We toured the ruins of Athens, the Acropolis citadel and the Parthenon temple. Later in Rome, Italy, we saw the ancient ruins of the Forum and the Colosseum. We went on to a tour of Ephesus, Turkey, where

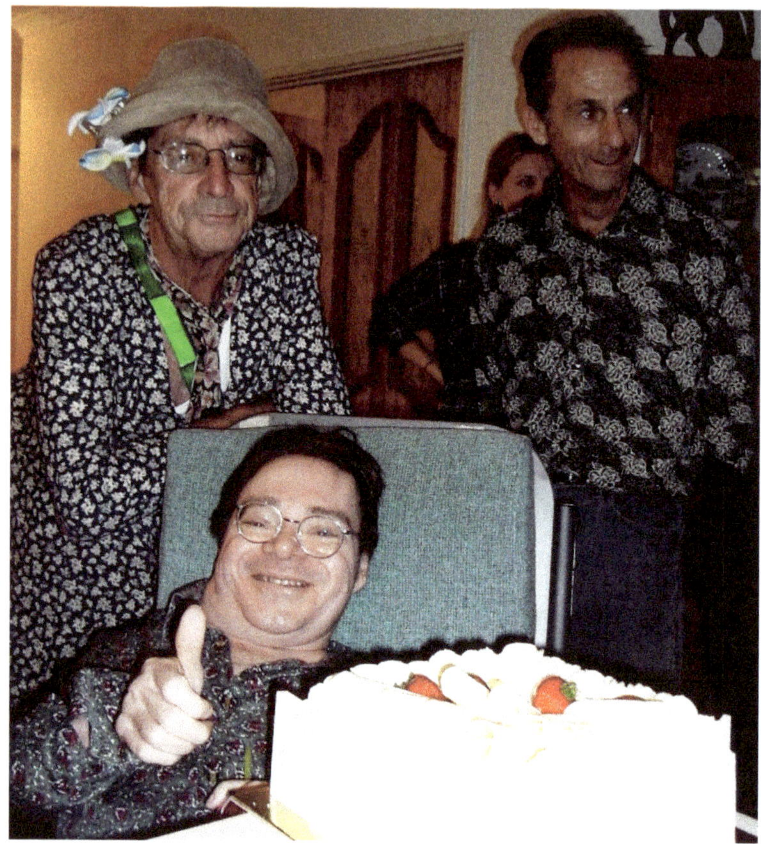

Stephen's birthday with Ray, the bag lady, and Stephen Upton, one of Steve's carers

Cleopatra and Mark Anthony had spent their honeymoon. It was amazing to us we could Skype Stephen from the other side of the world, showing him where we were.

On another long cruise with our friends Mick and Janet, we again furthered Stephen's knowledge through Skype. In Amsterdam after waiting in a long line, we went into the famous Anne Frank House where Anne and eight of her family members had hidden in the attic from the Nazis for two years. When discovered, the family had been sent to the concentration camps where Anne died a few weeks before World War II ended. Her father Otto survived.

We showed Stephen the Little Mermaid statue in Copenhagen and the beautiful Tivoli Gardens and amusement park. In Denmark, we went sightseeing on a hop-on-hop-off bus where Wi-Fi was available, so Stephen could see all the sites with us.

In Saint Petersburg, Russia, we toured the Church of the Savior on Spilled Blood and the Summer Palace of Peter the Great. We toured the Baltic Fountains at the Peterhof Palace, the Winter Palace, and the Hermitage, the home of Catherine the Great. The Hermitage is huge and to see all the exhibits treasured there is just impossible. It has been calculated that if you spend a minute at every item and eight hours in the Hermitage daily, it will take you almost 15 years to view all of the museum's exhibits.

To Stephen's delight we relayed the story of the famous Hermitage cats – a group of cats residing in the Hermitage Museum in Saint Petersburg, Russia. During the reign of Peter the Great, cats were brought into the museum to kill rats in the Winter Palace. The descendants of the cats living in the basement still occasionally wander through the Hermitage's courtyard and appear on the embankment and on the square during the summer. The museum has a press secretary dedicated to the cats and three people who act as caretakers.

Continuing on, we toured Helsinki, the capital of Finland; Tallinn, the capital of Estonia; and on to Stockholm, the capital of Sweden. Stephen needed many cushions for support to help him get comfortable when lying in bed. We were in a gift shop in Finland when I saw a 'moose' cushion, which would be perfect to support his knees.

Our friend Mick looked at me puzzled as I came out of the shop holding the cushion. "Why did you buy a stupid looking thing like that?"

Laughing at his expression, I explained it was exactly what Stephen needed for support under his legs.

"Oh," he said quietly.

I was grateful for sea days when we travelled by ship as we could rest and reflect upon all the places we had seen.

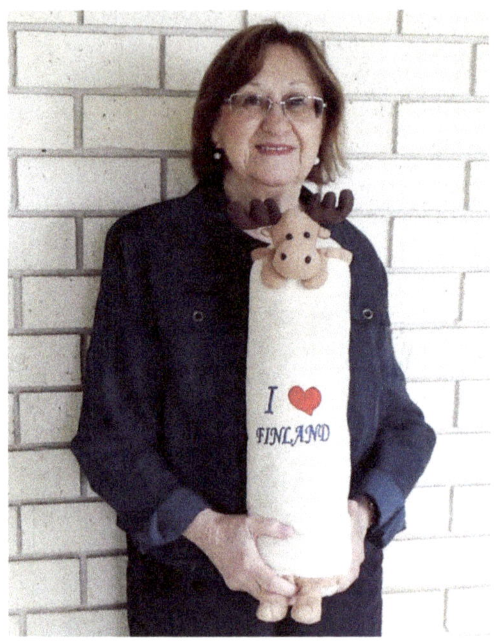

Me with the Moose pillow

In Norway, we went on to see the most beautiful scenery sailing through the Fjords. The magnificent scenery choked me up with emotion; it's something I will never forget. I was overjoyed and fulfilled that we could enhance Stephen's knowledge and enjoyment of the sites and history of so many exotic places.

We then boarded a train for sightseeing through Flam's mountains and waterfalls. We went on to Iceland and saw many small horses, learning they have two extra gaits. We saw more beautiful mountains and icebergs from our ship in Prince Christian Sound, Greenland, and stopped to see the local Inuit people and their way of life. We sailed on to St Johns, Newfoundland, and Halifax, Nova Scotia, where the graves of the victims of the Titanic can be seen in Fairview Lawn Cemetery.

We arrived in New York on the last part of our cruise just before sunrise. The Statue of Liberty was only just visible in the dark, but most moving was the silhouette of the skyscrapers as the sun rose.

Janet, Mick, Ray and I were walking around Times Square in New York when we came across a store Bubba Gump Shrimp Co – a derivative from Stephen's favourite movie Forrest Gump. We all charged inside, and Ray immediately took out his iPhone to Skype Steve to show him a tour around the shop. Due to some malfunction with the phone, Stephen could not hear his dad. Ray wanted Stephen to hang up the phone and try calling him again.

Janet and I were looking around at memorabilia when we suddenly heard Ray loudly yelling out several times: "Hang up the fucking phone!"

Everyone in the shop stopped to look around to see where the shouting was coming from. Janet and I knew it was Ray. Embarrassed, we quickly made for the front door exit, pretending we did not know this man having a meltdown in the store.

When Ray had stormed out of the shop, Janet and I hurriedly went back in to finish our souvenir shopping. We bought Steve a T-shirt.

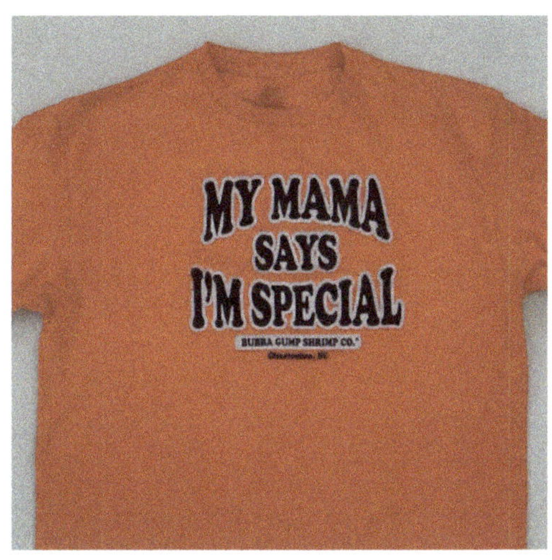

T-shirt from Bubba Gump Shrimp

Later, we were able to show Stephen on Skype the same scenery we were seeing of the city lights while riding around New York on a Wi-Fi enabled hop-on-hop-off bus. It was marvellous for Steve to be seeing this beautiful city at night the same time as us. It felt like he was with us on the bus. Steve could put our transmission on his 27-inch computer screen and be right there with us. We could see him and his carer, and they in turn could see us and the surrounding scenery.

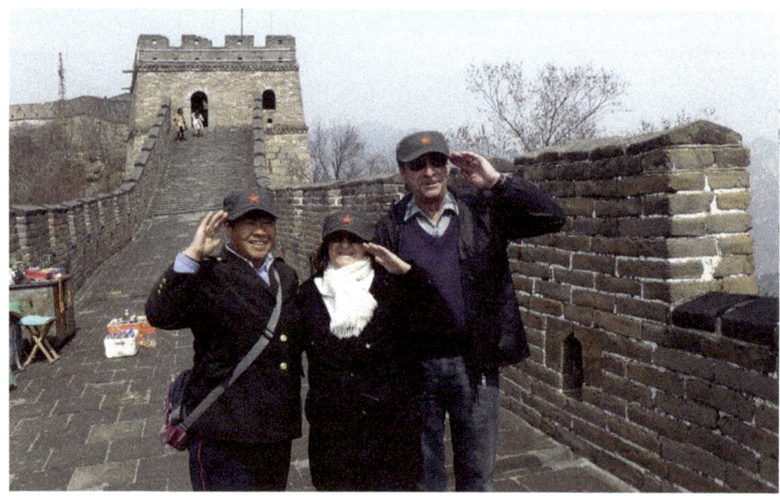

Guide and us on The Great Wall

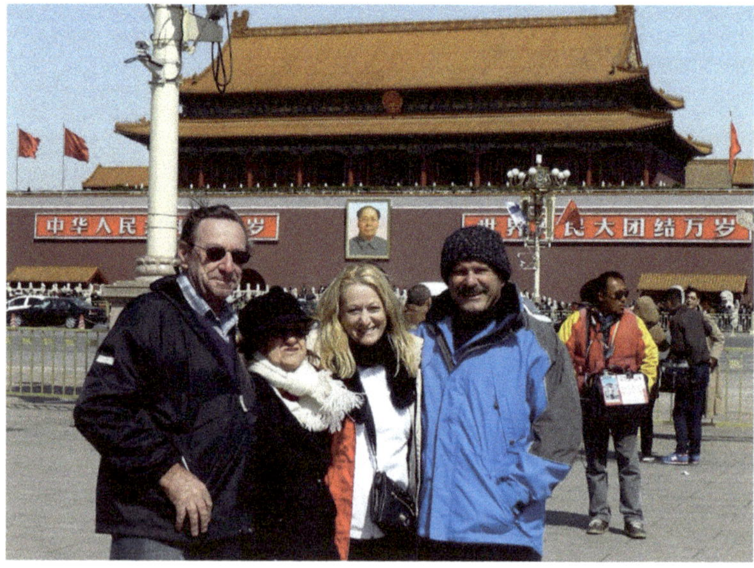

Ray, me, Janet and Mick at Tiananmen Square

Travelling on to Beijing, we successfully conquered a section of the Great Wall of China and marvelled at the story of its construction. The highlight of the visit was entering the fabled Forbidden City.

Arriving at Tiananmen Square, we saw with wonder that the vast area is dominated by a portrait of the late Chairman Mao. We made our way towards our destination, the Forbidden City. As we approached, with Ray trying in vain to connect to Stephen via Skype, we found the doors firmly closed as there was an 'important foreign visitor' – none other than the Australian Prime Minister – being given a private tour. Consequently, we never got to see inside.

Even though Stephen followed us everywhere through the internet and daily phone calls, our absence caused him much grief. His dedicated carers took care of all his needs; however, we knew Stephen was vulnerable. We were acutely aware that if anything happened to us while we were away, he was not in a position to manage his own care or take on the responsibilities of keeping a house. At times, it made him feel physically overwhelmed and helpless. We were burdened with guilt, but took comfort in knowing that we could show Stephen the world through our eyes and the internet. We knew the time would come when he would need to move into a facility, but none of us were ready to face this yet.

We decided we would once again go cruising with our good friends, Mick and Janet. We chose an Asian cruise from Hong Kong to Kobe and Nagasaki in Japan. We toured the Nagasaki Atomic Bomb Museum, next to which is the Nagasaki National Peace Memorial Hall dedicated to the victims of the atomic bomb.

With his iPhone, Ray Skyped Stephen, showing him the museum and Peace Park. Throughout Peace Park were statues donated by countries all over the world, symbolising peace and friendship. It is a reminder of World War II, a testament to the whole world striving for peace and friendship. Ray showed Stephen the exact place where America had dropped the atomic bomb. Standing there gave us a very sombre feeling. There was an abundance of overwhelming pictures and information of the destruction wrought on that tragic day, 9 August, 1945, at 11:02:35 AM.

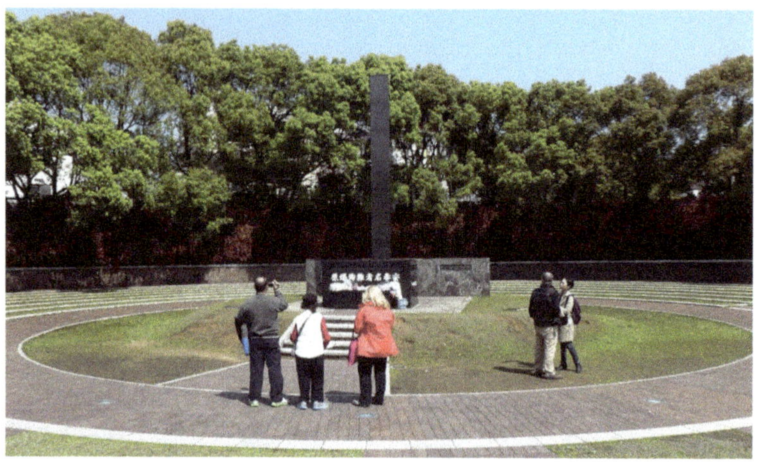

Mick, Janet and me where the atomic bomb hit

At home, Stephen had a pillow-and-sheet set with pictures of lions, tigers and giraffes. He took a photograph of these and showed his friends, comically claiming the pictures of these animals was from his own world travels during a safari trip. He had 'travelled' extensively with us via Skype with no passport required. Through us, he saw the world from his bed, which gave him an understanding of how the world worked.

Travelling, whether in person or by Skype, reassured him that the world is big, and gave him the strength to tolerate his frustrations and to deal with small-minded bureaucrats during the tough times ahead.

23

Disasters Strike

Somehow, good carers continued to turn up through all sorts of avenues. A government agency recommended a gentleman who was also called Stephen. To save confusion, we called our boy Steve or Stevie. Because Steve controlled his own funding, he employed Stephen Upton directly, until bureaucracy changed the rules and funding was managed by another organisation.

Stephen Upton arrived early for his interview as a carer and instantly connected with Steve. They shared a lot more in common than their first names. Stephen Upton recalls being shocked by Steve's physical appearance when he met Steve for the first time. "OI had bent his bones in cruel ways and made his limbs contracted and contorted." Yet he was impressed with Steve's wit and sense of humour, which was similar to his own.

Steve's carers had repeatedly told me his physical appearance quickly became unnoticeable once they spoke with him. They found him so easy to talk to, given his genuine interest in everyone and everything.

The pattern of Stephen Upton arriving early for work would continue for the next 13 years of faithful service. His reliability was second to none. No job was beneath him, and he had a quiet gentle way in which he humbly went about his work. It was amazing for me to have such good help and to know Steve was so well cared for.

Stephen Upton understood how authority could be misused, and how institutions could make silly blanket rules unsuitable for the individual's needs. This shared point of view connected him and Steve. All those years of serving Steve gave him insight into both humanity and inhumanity. "One of the funniest things was a certain human service that took over the management of Steve's funding. They wanted carers to use a hoist to lift him."

Stephen Upton refused to use the hoist because it put undue stress on Steve's bones causing stress fractures. It had more potential for harm than good.

"From the beginning, Steve trained me to lift him manually to his best advantage in both a comforting and caring manner. Steve and I also had in common that at one time we both had lived in the USA – me for 10 months and Steve for many years."

Stephen was one of the best carers Steve had. He remained a faithful friend for years later, and their friendship continued long after he left.

Bureaucracy and pain both hurt, one unnecessarily. The officials were unwavering on their 'no lift' policy. Countless meetings and arguments ensued about the hoist. They insisted it was necessary to save carers hurting their backs. Keep in mind Steve weighed just 42 lb or 19.5 kilograms. When I, who was less than five feet tall (152 cm) and suffered from OI myself, could lift Stephen, why couldn't anyone else?

We do need rules and structure to guide us, but their one-size-fits-all rules were inflexible and could become oppressive in nature. They did not consider Steve's individual needs. They would not listen to me, so I was totally powerless. They were working against us instead of with us.

Stephen would poke fun at the ridiculous 'no lift policy'. He once told Claire, "When a husband and wife get married and when the husband carries his wife over the threshold, I wonder if the Occupational Health and Safety Police would insist he use a hoist instead to carry out the manoeuvre?"

Due to the instability of his skeleton, Stephen did not want to be lifted by a hoist. The hoist's sling put unnecessary pressure on his fragile, fixed-position bones due to his frozen hip, which lacked the flexibility to mould to the shape of the sling. Still, the officials staunchly vowed their way was the only way. Stephen was forced to try something he and I knew would be detrimental to his wellbeing.

Stephen did not expect special treatment. He just asked for common sense in a rigid system that did not offer compassionate workarounds. Instead, they dug their heels in further, their hearts removed and replaced by clipboards and 45-page documents. They were not prepared to listen to Stephen in order to gain his trust, define the problem or talk about a solution. They stuck to their rules for nothing but stubbornness.

When he was unwillingly put into the sling of the hoist, it quickly became apparent to me that unnecessary fractures were imminent. I tried to stop them and reiterated how and why the hoist could inflict stress fractures to his frozen hip. Finally, they reluctantly conceded the hoist would not work. The organisation then devised the use of slide sheets to help Stephen in and out of bed. This old method was far less stressful on Stephen's body and safer to use than the hoist.

One day, Claire noticed Stephen's left ear was becoming very red and sore on the outside. His head was always inclined to the left side when lying in bed so he could see his computer. He would even work lying down, with the keyboard on his lap and the screen adjacent to him.

We had previously had many discussions with funding bodies who insisted he should be transferred by the hoist, but even then at 25 kg, he was still light enough to lift easily. The infamous and unusable hoist that was delivered to us was sitting dormant in our garage. One day, as Claire walked past the hoist, she stopped in her tracks struck by an idea.

"Can we connect the computer to the hoist, so it can be lowered and raised directly in front of you, keeping your head in a natural position?" she asked.

Stephen agreed. Claire's idea looked like it would work.

A friend drew up some plans, and Claire enlisted the help of her father and brother to build and attach a box to store computer gear in and

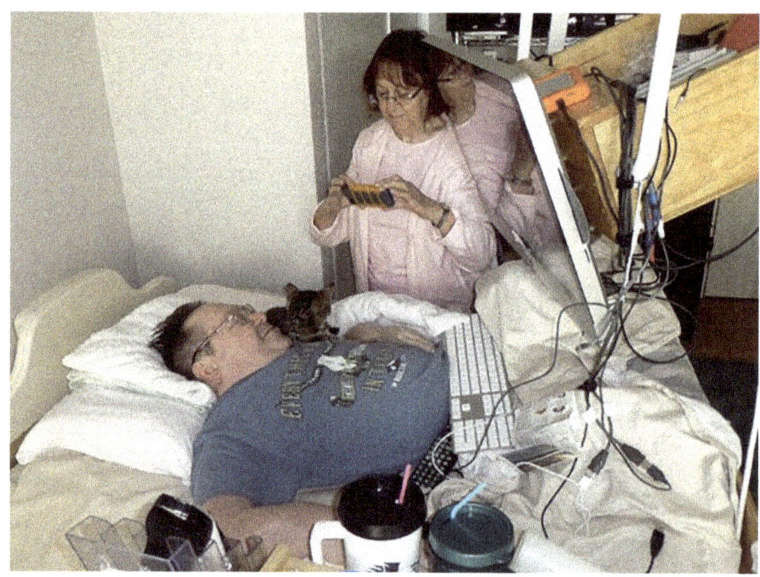

Me taking a photo of Stephen and Miffy

to design something for the screen to be attached to. Mathematical equations had to be worked out to calculate the hanging point of the box.

The day dawned for the hoist to be commissioned into its new role. The computer screen was attached and voila! – Stephen could see his computer without strain in a normal position, all thanks to Claire's ingenuity.

This was a significant improvement for Stephen. He could now use the computer without having to turn his head to the side. Something so simple made such a big difference for him.

'Time and tide wait for no man' says the old but true English adage. Ray's mother and Stephen's beloved Glasses Nana died aged 87. Ray's father followed three years later, aged 86, and our beloved Aunt Peggy departed at age 91, each leaving us sad but with many happy memories to find solace in.

It was about 9:15 PM one September night and I had just gone to bed. Ray went into Steve's room and asked him to put on the Bloomberg channel on his TV to see how the American stock markets were faring. That's when the news revealed a shocking sight of America under attack. Ray came to me and said, "Come and look at this! A plane just flew into the World Trade Centre and it's on fire."

We could not comprehend what we were seeing. We were overcome with extreme sadness for the people in the building. As the event unfolded, we saw a second plane hit the other tower. In utter horror and disbelief, we watched as the South Tower collapsed, followed by the announcement that a third plane had crashed into the Pentagon. A short time later, the North Tower collapsed too in yet another dust storm amidst tons of paper and debris flying everywhere. Terrified people were running away from the melee as fast as they could.

Then a fourth plane crashed into an empty field in Shanksville, Pennsylvania. Its target was to be the White House, but the terrorists on the plane had been overpowered by the brave passengers.

During the September 11 attacks in 2001, 2,996 people were killed (including the 19 hijackers) and more than 6,000 injured. These immediate deaths included the 265 people on the four planes (including the terrorists), the 2,606 people in the World Trade Centre and the surrounding area, and 125 people at the Pentagon.

We stayed up till morning watching the resulting chaos unfold. We went to bed near sunrise with many questions running through our heads. We had lived many years in America and loved it. This attack felt very personal.

A few weeks later, Stephen learned of the death of the Beatle, George Harrison, on 29 November, 2001, at age 58. Stephen fondly recalled how George and the The Traveling Wilburys had been the inspiration for his little band The Traveling Wheelchairies. George had written two of Stephen's favourite songs: 'My Sweet Lord' and 'Here comes the Sun'.

Soon after, Stephen complained of severe pain in his stomach. Upon admission to hospital, the doctors had him sign a form indicating he did not want to be resuscitated as was Stephen's wish. The doctors were able to clear his bowel without surgery, after which he was heavily sedated on a pain drip.

I was watching him when he suddenly stopped breathing. I quickly screamed for the doctors to come. They came straightaway but said, "He does not want to be resuscitated."

"No, no, no!" I screamed in alarm. "He does want to be resuscitated; he just doesn't want his chest compressed as that would break his ribs!"

Understanding dawned on their faces. They told me to wait outside because what they were going to do would upset me further. I paced past the glass doors and telephoned Ray, who was working on a mine 110 miles away. Thank God, he answered me straightaway! Between sobs, I said, "Ray, come quickly to the hospital. We are losing Stephen! He stopped breathing and they are working on him."

"I'm leaving now," was all he said before hanging up.

I proceeded to telephone Claire and Chris, Stephen's carer, to come to the hospital.

Claire left work and drove in such a stressed and dazed state that she got lost. Due to her worry, she couldn't remember where the hospital was, despite having visited it on multiple occasions. Nevertheless, she arrived before Ray, who broke several speed limits and turned up in his mining clothes and muddy boots. I was so relieved to see him. The hospital staff reluctantly let him through their clean sterilised ward to Stephen's bedside.

Ray joined Claire and me at the bedside. Stephen, now awake, looked up at Ray and weakly muttered a greeting. Ray could see Stephen was feeling extremely uncomfortable and quickly realised he had messed in his bed. When Stephen was unconscious, his muscles relaxed, including those that control the bladder and bowel. Ray leaned forward and lifted Stephen clear off the bed to enable the nurses to clean Stephen and replace the bed linen. When everything was clean, Ray placed Stephen carefully back on his bed.

The crisis now over, Ray reassured Stephen he would be okay. Then with a hug and much handshaking, Ray drove back to work at a much-reduced pace.

Stephen's daily care thereafter became more labour intensive.

Why would anyone want to read about a laborious toileting procedure, you ask? I say it is a golden opportunity to remind ourselves to be grateful of our independence while we have it. Simple activities such as toileting were a mammoth effort for Stephen.

The pain medication Stephen used intermittently caused constipation. If Stephen were to strain while going to the toilet, it could result in coccyx fracture or a prolapse of the bowel. Both of these episodes had happened previously, during which time he had remained calm and humorous as always. We had become experts at fixing the prolapse by gently applying pressure to the area for a few seconds until the bowel returned to its rightful position.

With all the straining in the toilet, Stephen developed a very painful thrombosed haemorrhoid. With crisis nine hundred and ninety-nine looming overhead, I called his doctor who was reluctant to treat him at home. Despite my pleas, he advised that Stephen should go to the hospital. He was oblivious to the rigmarole a hospital visit entailed. We would need to take Stephen's own special pillows, his own commode, a special pressure mattress, his medications… and on the list goes. Plus there was the risk of fractures when moving him around the hospital, which meant explaining to everyone how to handle Stephen. Frankly, the whole process of going to the hospital was unnecessary and exhausting for Stephen.

I called Claire, who was by then a fully trained Registered Nurse, and explained the scenario. She came at once to help.

In her words she reiterated later:

"Fortunately, I had some limited medical equipment at home that I could use to help Stephen. I was shaking on the inside as I used the scalpel without the luxury of a local anaesthetic to numb the area and prevent pain. I was terrified of the risks of infection or making him septic while in bed. As I cut into the area Stephen did not flinch but remained cheerful and stoic. Not even the slightest whimper came from him. I guess he was so used to pain that it was not a new experience for him. I removed the large clot whilst murky waters of self-doubt threatened to drown my rapidly spiralling self-confidence. With the clot excised, Stephen experienced immediate relief and was extremely grateful.

"Heather then went on to thank me for helping and told me I was so calm throughout the ordeal. Little did she know that on the inside I had been shaking, scared and frightened throughout – and for days afterwards I continued to worry that an infection would develop. However, the area healed, the persistent ache resolved and an unnecessary trip to hospital was avoided, and all ended well."

Stephen's doctor advised that the use of a suppository would stop him having to strain himself. Initially, carers were not permitted to insert the suppositories due to bureaucratic red tape. An external agency had to be employed at significant financial cost to insert the suppositories. After many fights and wringing of hands with the officials and their silly rules, the carers were trained by nurses to insert suppositories themselves.

As time passed, Stephen's spine was no longer strong enough for him to sit up for any period of time. He was unable to use a household toilet, so he had to be laid down on his commode with a basin of water underneath.

Although getting out of bed caused Stephen pain and discomfort, it provided a much-needed chance for his lungs to drain any excess collection that might have occurred whilst lying flat. While he was in the bathroom, the carer remade his bed to look inviting with clean sheets.

Stephen made jokes about his situation and made all of us laugh even in despair. He intuitively knew how to see the funny side of any dismal situation. We taught him that.

24

Policy, Power, Politics

Stephen continued to have control of his own funding for his care. He hired the carers and paid them from funds distributed to him by the government. He ran a simple computer program to keep a tally of his carer's wages. Everything ran in perfect harmony until it was strongly suggested that Stephen have an agency run the operation for him to save time, trouble and paperwork. They promised they would be able to recruit staff to help him manage his current funds and provide various other supports – too good to be true!

I sensed that something was not right. My intuition proved to be correct. Bumbledom, or the officious and pompous behaviour of minor officials and its associated misery, describes the situation perfectly. Stephen's path changed with enforced bureaucracy causing endless frustration and repetition of useless tasks.

After the battle with the hoist, the officials began to enforce new rules about Stephen's pain medication. They told him he must manage all aspects of his pain pills himself. They did not want any involvement because some medications had an opiate base. They insisted that his medication must be supplied from the pharmacy weekly in a sealed plastic package, which was exceedingly difficult for him to pry open with his thin, weak fingers.

All this without any acknowledgment of the fact that Stephen was disabled and in pain. It would have been simple for them to help keep him comfortable without taking legal responsibility; yet they coldheartedly refused to help him with his medication.

Then came hyper-vigilance as the agency ensured no one was breaking the rules. Carers were not allowed to help him with the very medication that was so important for his pain control and which he needed most. Other types of medication could be administered by carers; however, they were not to be handled without wearing gloves. What would happen if they touched it, I wondered. Was it going to blow up or explode? It was protocol gone mad, as I saw it.

In the event that a pain pill was dropped, the carers were told not to administer the pill but to destroy it, and then write an incident report and inform their superiors of their actions. In the meantime, Stephen would be in pain while the carer awaited further instructions from the supervisor. How ridiculous!

This rampant stupidity created a culture of fear among the carers, who had to comply with rules in order to keep their employment. The very organisation that was supposed to take care of Stephen had created a philosophy of anxiety for him and his carers. Being disabled, Stephen was unable to physically handle his medications and needed my help every day.

I researched other organisations to see how they handled medications for their clients. Ironically, they allowed carers to give the same medication to patients who were intellectually disabled, but our organisation had a neurotic desire to assert control. Stephen even offered to sign a legal waiver to say they were absolved from taking any clinical responsibility for the administration of his medication, but the agency stood rigid and firm. Being as vulnerable as he was, Stephen had no choice but to accept their rulings.

I saw red when their 'brightest authoritarian' approached Stephen and said, "Your world is so small, Mr Simpson. Do you know you take 27 tablets per day?"

Stephen with respect and good manners just smiled back politely, while I raged inside at their judgement and insensitivity.

With their brains working overtime, the bureaucrats came up with more 'brilliant' ideas:

Carers could hand him his medication pack, but were not allowed to touch or open it – the exact help he most needed. We were told we could hire a nurse to administer his pills. Keep in mind this would be necessary all hours throughout the day and the night and at our expense, just to satisfy their rules.

As part of their repertoire of extreme brilliance, they brought in a small device for Stephen to open the blister pack of pills. I'm all for helping people to be independent, but it was a ludicrous solution. The device needed two working hands and for the person to be able to sit upright – neither of which Stephen could do with his weak spine and one semi-useable arm.

The bureaucrats prioritised their rules, without a thought for Stephen's needs. There was no kindness or empathy in their hearts to even consider an exception to their rules. Their instructions had to be obeyed at all costs.

At the same time, I would get frequent phone calls saying they did not have a carer for Steve that day. They would contact another agency but if no one was available, I would have to take over myself. One of my old beloved carers would help if they could, but inevitably I was left on my own.

To solve this problem, they had another 'brainwave'. They sent a carer who would be a mentor and trainer for new carers. The senselessness of this was I had to first show the mentor the care procedures needed for Stephen in order for the mentor to train new carers. Stephen and I would laugh our heads off at their comedy of errors of Tweedledum and Tweedledee.

We had well-meaning substitute carers who had their own ideas about how to cure Stephen's ailment. One was earnest about herbal medicine and a crystal lamp that would rid the air of negative ions for relieving his pain. If only it was that easy, there would be no painful diseases left in the world. Nevertheless, I rushed out and purchased the magic lamp to please him, but sadly nothing changed.

Later, when new carers applied confessing they had no previous training or experience, I would tell them, "Great! Come on in. You don't need any!"

Stephen knew untrained workers were often better because their hearts were still soft, trainable and sympathetic. They had not become bitter and cynical from compassion fatigue or addicted to obeying rules.

In order to show us they were such good providers, the dictators made up pages and pages of documents containing questions and answer choices for Stephen to fill in regarding his care. Given Stephen was lying on his back with little mobility, one can only imagine how difficult and tiresome it was for him. Looking at these survey sheets, Stephen would often laugh and say, "Give me strength!" I would assist him to fill in pages of futile questions that were not even relevant to his condition. Instead of taking five minutes to listen to us to solve our problems, they gave us twenty days' worth of inane and unhelpful paperwork. It was an exercise in futility and made a mockery of Stephen's needs.

Stephen did not need any of this; he needed compassion and understanding. They took away his basic rights. They were horrible human beings with no heart or soul, only interested in power and control and their paperwork. In my opinion, the followers of bureaucrats' rules should have communicated with the rule makers to sort out the many exceptions to their directives, but I suppose that would have taken 100 years of useless meetings to find a solution.

It was all too much for me. I was driving along the freeway one day when it occurred to me that I didn't know who I was or where I was going. I tried to look in my handbag for a clue of some kind that might jog my memory, but I could not find anything. I tried not to panic, thinking that is if I came across a hospital I would go in and seek help. After driving around for half an hour looking for a hospital, I came across a street that I recognised and suddenly I knew who I was and where I was going.

Apparently, I was under so much stress from dealing with bureaucrats and their many pointless protocols, policies and procedures that I had had an episode of amnesia, shutting my mind down to reality. It was alarming and weird and very scary.

Ray and I were very worried as to how our boy's future would be, given he was in declining health with his pain becoming more unmanageable, and the fact that we were not getting any younger. If something were to happen to us, I wondered how Stephen would cope with our large house. Since he was confined to his bed 90 percent of the time, he would not know what was happening beyond his room.

The war between the administrators and us became more intense and ridiculous. They made Stephen's life and ours a living hell.

I found an organisation for Stephen that would provide temporary accommodation from his present predicament. I was delighted to learn there was a spa bath which had been generously installed due to funding efforts. Thinking it would do wonders for Stephen's therapy, I happily agreed for him to stay for a short time. I had previously drawn up a list of his daily needs and the care requirements that carers had to follow, making it easier for him and everybody involved.

At first, everyone seemed willing to make his time amicable and happy, but soon after, neglect became more and more apparent. Needless to say, without my watchful eye, Stephen's personal care diminished together with the same old political issues to contend with.

Stephen was reluctant to tell me they had left him on the toilet unattended for 80 minutes. With his iPhone, he telephoned their office several times. Eventually someone answered, and only then was Stephen helped with the toilet and shower. It took many days to relieve his added back pain resulting from sitting on the toilet for so long.

On another occasion when I went to visit him, he had a terrible rash on his head and neck from not having been showered regularly, and his bed was sopping wet from perspiration. When I complained angrily about this neglected hygiene, their shoddy excuse was they thought he had been sleeping and did not want to wake him, so they had left him all day in this deplorable condition.

After that episode, I would visit daily to make sure Stephen was being well cared for.

I found that the spa bath was never used by Stephen or any other residents. No one was permitted to lift Stephen in and out of the spa because of their bureaucratic rules. The only thing that had touched the inside of the spa was dust. How sad and disappointed I was at the whole farcical respite situation.

Then they had the audacity to give me an invoice for the worthless, traumatic time Stephen had endured there.

I was outraged with the gross negligence when Steve was in respite. I was sad and dejected about his poor care, intertwined with endless bureaucracy. My heart broke for my dear boy – no lover, no legs, no life, just putting up with imbecilic bureaucracy treating him like an idiot and ruling his life.

After Stephen came home from respite, I began to investigate other organisations as options. I wanted Stephen to have the best care possible. Unfortunately, each potential agency had the same bureaucratic rules regarding the use of a hoist and Stephen's care.

When our organisation discovered we were looking elsewhere, they applied to the government for more funding to continue providing care for Stephen and requested astronomical amounts. They insisted Stephen sign their forms for more funding at their convenience, by even barging into the toilet when he was trying to have a bowel motion. They explained they did not have time to wait for him to finish – as if they were highly important people!

To add salt to the wound, within days they repeated this invasion of his privacy on two more occasions.

Stephen's sanity was saved from these frustrations by his old friend John.

Because Stephen would be busy during the day with his carers and his care routine, he would often wake up in the middle of the night or early morning to pursue his interests such as connecting with friends, listening to music and doing intellectual internet searches. His computer was a lifeline of information for him.

One night, during Stephen's personal time, his phone rang. It was 1:00 AM. Wondering who could be calling him at this hour, Stephen answered.

"I knew the only person who would be awake at one in the morning would be Stephen Simpson," said a familiar voice from his past. It was John, Stephen's friend from the nursing home. Stephen was pleasantly surprised.

John explained he was not happy with a painting he was doing and had decided to cover it up with white paint and start again. The white paint was dripping down in a way that reminded him of foam on a wave. He was so happy when he finished the painting of barrelling waves that he wanted to tell someone about the explosion of ideas he had had when completing this masterpiece, and had thought of Stephen.

Immediately John and Stephen reconnected, reciting Monty Python skits that each knew word for word. Together they lampooned the bureaucratic rules they had to live by. They saw the funny side in overcoming adversity together. They laughed about the time when they had first become acquainted in the care facility.

John, who was new then at the facility, had been moved to a room opposite Stephen's. Stephen was playing music at 2:00 AM when John was trying to sleep. He asked the carer to turn off the music. When John met Stephen the next day, he warned him that if Stephen played his music again so late at night when he was trying to sleep, he would burn Stephen's Beatle albums that were on top of his stereo.

Stephen just said, "Okay."

Each day at breakfast, Stephen and his group of close friends in wheelchairs would always joke about anything and everything to distract themselves from the circumstances of their lives. John and Stephen had become good friends sharing each other's humour as well as music. Before John's disability, he had been a musician, singing and playing his guitar in a band.

Now that John had connected with Stephen again, he reached out to Stephen and helped him through depression. John made many visits to Stephen now living with us. John told me he had endured his own depression with Stephen's help and company.

On one of these visits, John recalled how a carer he had had from another organisation had mentioned knowing a guy who had brittle bones. John asked surprised, "Stephen Simpson? You know him?" The carer went on to tell John how amazed she had been by Stephen's happy, creative and supportive personality in spite of his situation. She had been strongly affected simply by the person that Stephen was.

25

A Little Help From Friends

John and Stephen talked daily with each other, bantering back and forth with their shared sense of humour. They philosophised and talked at length about movies they could relate to, given their own circumstances. Being homebound, Stephen loved watching movies and television – the realizations he had from his favourite movies and shows gave great meaning to the world around him, thereby shaping his existence.

The character of Nurse Ratched in the movie One Flew over the Cuckoo's Nest represented to Stephen a nurse with a cold heartless tyrannical fanaticism for controlling her environment. Stephen and John had encountered individuals with these personalities. People in authority often advised carers against getting too close to their client. I cannot imagine how these people can order someone not to have feelings, can you? "It is soul crushing and illogical. It goes past tragedy and comes back around as comedy," was Stephen's interpretation. Sadly, I too have observed people with such traits in high-ranking positions.

The movie I am Sam was special to Stephen because the main character Sam was obsessed with the Beatles. The soundtrack has many Beatles songs. In the movie, Sam has a seven-year-old daughter he names Lucy Diamond after the Beatles song. Lucy is born to a homeless woman who leaves the scene soon after, leaving Lucy with her father who has the mind of a seven-year-old. As Lucy grows older and surpasses her father mentally, the authorities decide she would be better off with foster parents who would be better able to raise her into adulthood. Stephen loved this film for its simple message – that all you need is love – and felt the whole world could benefit from being reminded of its meaning.

In my own situation with my boy, I had the mental capacity to not only deal with the many problems in raising Stephen, but also to love him unconditionally. It was all I needed to get him through to manhood and beyond.

Stephen acquired courage and wisdom through his pain, and faith and hope through his suffering. He stood firmly by the Golden Rule: Do unto others as you would have them do unto you. Needless to say, Stephen applied his wisdom to help others with their various predicaments, and so he made many close friends.

With time, the burden of policies and procedures lightened through discreet compromises without breaking any rules, making for a more harmonious environment.

As Ray and I were both approaching our senior years, we again began thinking more about Stephen's future care should something happen to us. We were conscious of needing to have Stephen settled in a good place, in the event of our sudden demise.

After exhaustingly re-searching many places and after many interviews, I found a facility caring for people with cerebral palsy. They were expanding and looking into taking in people with other disabilities. They seemed to fully understand our predicament and Stephen's ongoing care and accommodation requirements.

Stephen was very anxious and fearful about moving from his home. He frequently shouted at us. I completely understood his frustration and helplessness. I would run up to the remotest room in the house just to cry with all the pain in my heart. I consoled myself with thoughts that he was at least exercising his lungs during these angry outbursts. One of his carers told me he had said, “My parents don’t want to look after me anymore.”

I was devastated one minute and angry the next at his cutting choice of words. Weren’t we doing the best we could for him? But then I would put myself in his place and feel his behaviour was completely warranted. Whenever these unhappy episodes occurred, Ray would remain calm and simply make a cup of tea for Steve.

With calm restored, Ray explained to Steve the possible situation of both of us being killed in an accident; he would be left alone in our large house, unable to manage even the simplest household chores. The prospect was daunting and the financial requirements of maintaining the house and gardens were completely beyond Stephen’s capabilities. Eventually, Steve accepted the reasoning behind our decision to move him.

We all made several trips to Stephen’s new home to assess the best way to set up his room. We purchased a set of shelving for his stereo and television, and I asked for many more power outlets to be installed, in order to operate all his equipment.

The day arrived when we packed Stephen’s music gear and belongings into a moving truck. Chris, Steve’s carer, helped us load all belongings into the truck. We all arrived at a lovely home just 20 minutes’ drive from ours.

Stephen was given the biggest room across from a large bathroom at the back of the house. The bathroom could easily accommodate wheelchairs and even wet beds for showering, depending on the clients' physical disabilities.

We were greeted by four carers: brothers Peter and John, Rupinda, and Rinku. They did everything they could to help Stephen be comfortable in his new home. They were also welcoming to Stephen's friend Claire, allowing her to stay overnight with her bedding and to sleep on the floor beside his bed.

Peter and John had a witty sense of humour, providing the normality that Stephen craved. They laughed a lot together and their comradeship was simply genuine. Peter and John provided communication and practical help in parallel and in direct contrast with the so-called experts, many of whom charged very high sums for very little in return.

John helped set up Stephen's computer onto the hoist and connected the electrical cords intertwined with his television and music equipment. Peter, meanwhile, cut a sleeve off one of his own cotton jumpers making a kind of holder for Stephen's left thigh, which had recently sustained a stress fracture and needed a support brace. The sleeve fitted perfectly and added extra comfort and support. No task was too hard for them. They were always willing to help Stephen with whatever he needed and were skilled at thinking outside the square to solve any challenges.

Stephen was using his right arm a lot. Over time it became very sore and we suspected his arm had a stress fracture. Claire arranged an in-centre visit with the physiotherapist who had previously made the support splint for his left thigh. He came to see Stephen at the facility, so he could make the splint for his arm without Stephen having to leave his bed.

I was called aside by management to tell me that Stephen should have been taken to the hospital, and that I should not have planned myself to have the splint made. I explained to the powers-that-be that I had simply fixed the problem without rounding up his medications, taking all his support pillows and personal commode, lifting him several times for unnecessary X-rays, and explaining to all new persons his condition and how to take care of him. Their rules would have made Stephen wait in pain while they managed the many phone calls, meetings and arranging for his essentials to accompany him to the hospital.

Still they insisted that their rules should have been adhered to. Again, bureaucracy hurt more than helped.

Vera, a lovely woman, did most of the cooking for the residents. She made many of Stephen's favourite meals for him. Her sincerity in caring for Stephen and others was genuine and heart-warming to see.

While visiting Stephen one day, I walked into the kitchen. I noticed Vera talking to a girl with cerebral palsy sitting beside her at a table while she was writing records into the house notebook. I was amazed at Vera having a conversation with the young girl who was only able to make certain sounds.

Most of the other residents were entirely mute as a result of cerebral palsy, but the carers knew how to communicate with everyone. These carers were all very gifted, giving everything to the clients and their work.

Stephen, as was his nature, entertained everyone with his music, wit and endless stories of travels from our time in America. The carers were enchanted listening to his adventures and watching Google Earth to see every road and highway he had travelled. He had a remarkable memory. To their amazement, he could tell them the time, day and place of his every adventure.

It was wonderfully relieving to see Stephen happy in his new home. We laughed so much when a young girl with cerebral palsy who could talk wanted to visit Stephen in his room for company and conversations. Stephen was exhausted talking with her for hour on end, and had asked her to call out to him first in case he may be asleep.

"Steve, are you awake?" she would ask.

"Nooo," Stephen would answer.

Cats always played a big part in Stephen's life. He always found great comfort in a cat's loyalty and friendship. I asked if I could introduce a kitten into the home, explaining that the presence of a house cat would be beneficial for everyone. The carers were a bit puzzled about this idea at first, but after thinking about it, they agreed. I remembered back when Stephen was in another institution, he had not been allowed to have a cat. The reason being bureaucracy's rules declared that cats were unhygienic.

There was one challenge though. The cat needed to be allergy free as one of the residents was allergic to cats. After much research, we found a cute one in Adelaide (2,700 km. away), and were more than prepared to pay for the cost of the cat and to have it transported to Perth. Just as we were about to pay, we looked the phone number up on Google and found it was a scam. To rip anyone off is appalling, but to rip someone off for buying a cat as a companion for the disabled – that is just truly despicable.

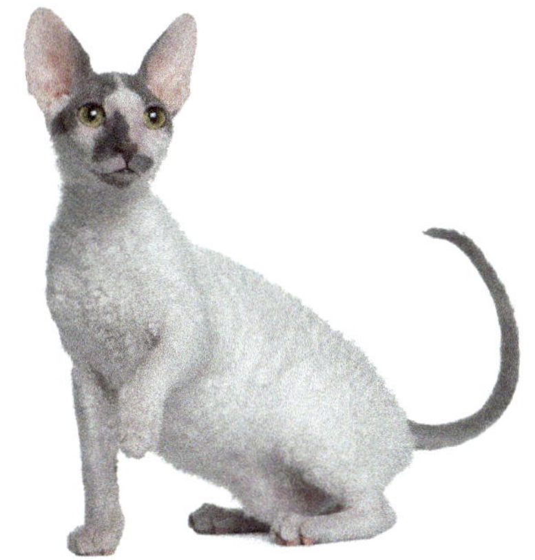

I made some local enquires and acquired a lovely little tabby rescue kitten named Miffy. I took her to show Stephen and the other residents. Their faces lit up with 1000-watt smiles. Even though most residents could not use words, their excitement was evident on their faces. One resident in particular had involuntary spontaneous reflexes that he simply had no control over. I carefully placed Miffy on his shoulder. Unfortunately, his arm had a spasm and accidentally struck Miffy quite hard on her head. Miffy did not flinch. She calmly stayed put. It was as if she knew she had a special role as a 'therapy cat' to play in providing comfort to this boy.

Another time, I sat Miffy near the feet of a girl in her wheelchair and proceeded to walk back to Stephen's room. I was away just a short time and when I came back, Miffy was still sitting where I had put her. It was wonderful to see the wide smile on the girl's face as she giggled with glee. Miffy was indeed the best companion for everyone living in Stephen's new home.

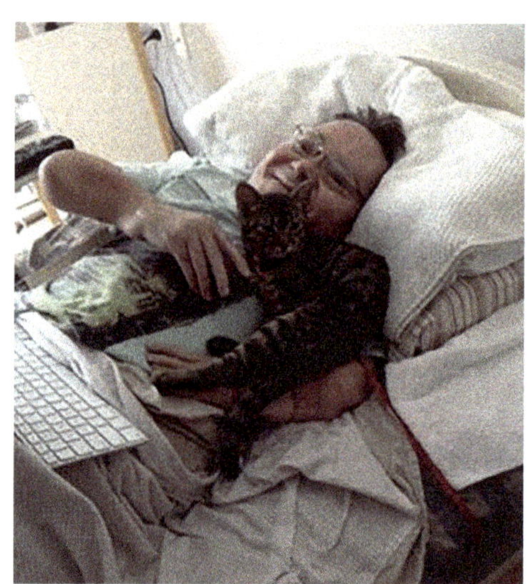

Stephen and Miffy

Stories are now abundant about the benefits of animals for the sick and disabled in nursing homes, and the value of therapy dogs travelling with their owners can be seen in airports all over the world.

After Stephen was happy and settled into his new home, I thought about going to see the Calgary Stampede in Calgary, Canada, something I had always wanted to see. Ray booked our flights and accommodation straightaway. Stephen was not happy about us leaving again however, I was satisfied he would be well looked after and comforted by the carers in our absence.

The ten-day event was beyond all my expectations. I was thrilled every minute with the bucking horses and huge cows, the cutting horse trials and the chuck wagon races. I was utterly in my domain. I thought about my father being in Canada when he was a young man, captivated by the cowboy lifestyle, as I have been. With a smile, I imagined him doing his rope tricks at the Calgary Stampede.

The latest model cars and Winnebagos were either for sale or drawn as prizes in various raffles daily. We wondered how we would get home the Corvette, my favorite car, if we won it, and finally decided not to buy the $5 ticket. The final night's fireworks entertainment was spectacular, and we went to our motel almost walking on air. My lifetime dream of attending the Calgary Stampede was better than I had ever imagined.

We went on a long train ride through the Rocky Mountains on the famous Rocky Mountaineer train. We saw the most beautiful scenery of mountains, glaciers and lakes in Banff National Park and Lake Louise. We saw wildlife such as deer, moose, mountain goats, bighorn sheep and black bears. At Jasper National Park, our guide told an interesting story of Mount Edith Cavell, a mountain located in the valleys of Jasper National Park.

The mountain was named in 1916 for Edith Cavell, an English nurse executed by the Germans during the Great War for having helped Allied soldiers escape from occupied Belgium to the Netherlands. Cavell's remains were returned to Britain after the war. Overlooking Trafalgar Square is a monument dedicated to brave Edith Cavell.

While on the train, everyone was asked to write a note describing what we had seen. Ray wrote a poem. To our delight, he won first prize with a small pin entitled Order of the Salmon.

I wish I were an Engineer
Aboard the Rocky Mountaineer,
Helping people just like you,
Enjoy the ever-changing view
People here with eager faces
From far and wide, exotic places
From far across the raging seas,
You come and visit sights like these,
Over there a female moose
Rubs against a leafy Spruce
And to your left a grizzly bear
Ambles slowly without care
While from his lofty perch on high
A mountain goat counts passers-by
Every several miles it seems
We are crossing raging streams
Everywhere it's verdant green
Environmentally a dream
And if my work career I've missed
I've crossed this off my Bucket List
In closing let me make it clear
I love the Rocky Mountaineer.

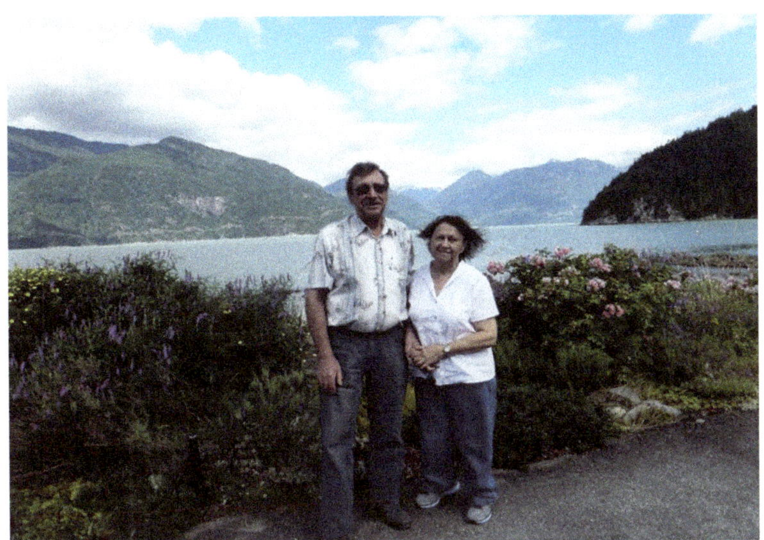

On one of our tours in beautiful Vancouver

26

All You Need Is Love

Ray and I returned from our overseas holiday early on the morning of Wednesday, August 13, 2014. We had been away for several weeks and were anxious to see our boy and spend time with him. As soon as we had been cleared from customs and had arrived home, I quickly unpacked a remote-control toy helicopter I had purchased for him while on our travels. I knew he was going to have a lot of fun with it.

When we arrived, he had a visitor and since they were chatting on merrily about music, we chose not to interrupt, but told him we would be back and left the helicopter with him.

The following day we went back to see Stephen. He had a bone scan scheduled. He told me he did not want the scan, but I encouraged him to get it done. I was anxious to see if his skeleton had improved. We knew how much pain our travelling caused him, and he was not looking forward to having his fragile skeleton put at risk to more pain and possibly a broken bone.

The hospitals had a no lift policy, and a hoist transfer increased the risk of fractures. A bone scan always involved him having to take along his own carer who knew how to lift him and place him gently on the hard table in order to have the procedure. In this case, Chris was going to take him. I felt happy he was in good hands.

I promised Stephen that we would get his computer fixed to give him something to take his mind off the scan, which was always very trying for him. His computer, his lifeline to the outside world, had been very unreliable of late and caused him much anxiety and stress when it would not function correctly.

Later, after Stephen was back from the scan, we spoke with John who said he was exhausted after the scan and that he had a lot of phlegm and was now sleeping.

The following day, Claire got a call from one of the carers saying, "Stephen is acting strangely. He is very confused. He told me he felt like his arm was not attached to his body."

Claire did not know what was wrong and told the carer to inform us and call an ambulance that Friday afternoon. When the ambulance arrived and the paramedics asked Stephen what they could do to help, Stephen in a daze said, "Can you fix my computer for me?"

Stephen was taken to the emergency ward and we immediately drove to the hospital. We found Stephen saturated in pools of sweat and his eyes bulging. When he looked at me, I could see sheer terror in his eyes, which frightened me to the core. He was a lot different from just a few days ago.

He smiled weakly and kept asking me to push the pillow up under his legs, even though the pillow was already present; in his state, he could not feel it there. We repeatedly reassured him the pillow was there, but he went on asking us to push it up to support his leg. Strangely, he did not even ask for pain relief medication, something he had been taking day in and day out.

Once Stephen was admitted, the doctors called us aside to talk about our options. It was a given that Stephen was not a suitable candidate for CPR. Compressions would just crush his chest. However, they could insert a tube into him which would connect to a special machine to help him breathe, but it wasn't necessarily a curative intervention; it might just prolong the inevitable.

This was frightening news and we felt terribly helpless and afraid. I implored, "He doesn't want to die, but he wouldn't want to live like that."

I did not want him to suffer, but I did not want to lose him either. Even though I had heard what the doctors said, I had not really comprehended what they were trying to tell me. It was impossible for me to take it in. They looked at me as if I was not getting their message. My throat felt constricted and my breathing became rapid and difficult. I was hyperventilating, too distraught for either words or breath. The twin burdens of shock and sorrow had enveloped me in a cloak of enormous weight.

Despite our grief, deciding not to opt for a ventilator appeared to be the kindest choice, and I feel our decision was to the doctor's relief.

Later, Claire made a surprise visit and sneakily ambled into his hospital room with her iPhone. Stephen had mentioned when she brought her iPhone earlier to get a special protective lens cover put on it. She wanted to capture their happy reunion with his familiar beautiful smile when he first saw her. Little did she know the lens cover was 'on' the iPhone at the time, preventing any photos.

We were surprised to see Claire, and a joyous big smile spread across Stephen's face. Nasal prongs were delivering him oxygen, but he did not appear to have any breathing difficulties as he saw her.

"C-l-a-i-r-e!!" he called out, spelling her name phonetically. Claire was so pleased to see him, they spent an hour of unadulterated bliss and basked in the presence of someone who genuinely loved and accepted the other, foibles and all. They reminisced about old times and we all laughed heartily.

Meanwhile, the standard hospital delicacy was delivered for Stephen's lunch: unappetizing overcooked vegetables and dry fish. Ray took one look and remarked, "Ahhh, I see we are having lobster again today."

Claire offered to feed Stephen, and graciously he accepted. After giving him a few spoonfuls, she discovered he was holding it in his cheeks as he did not have the energy to eat and simply was not hungry – but he didn't want to hurt her feelings by saying no. Characteristically he did not complain. He always wanted to be the best patient.

Stephen looked relatively well in Claire's company. His spirit was lively and his humour mischievous. Claire had a long drive home, so she reluctantly left his bedside but reassured him she would be back super soon.

As she headed out of his room and down the corridor, she could hear him saying repeatedly, "Goodbye Claire, goodbye." His voice floated down the hospital corridor, enveloping her in deep sadness, but she consoled herself with the fact she would see him again. She knew her boy was a survivor.

Some things Stephen fervently desired in life were:

He wanted nurses and doctors to have genuine and friendly relationships with their patients. The word 'nurse' means to hold, and Stephen was aware there were many ways to 'hold' someone, both physical or spiritual. The ironic thing was Stephen supported many others by nursing them along through their sorrows.

He wanted to facilitate a cultural change within nursing to encourage nurses to build genuine and empathetic relationships with their patients. He saw the best nurse as someone who would do anything to make her patient comfortable, would spend time for chats and share a sense of humour.

A doctor is a person who is qualified to treat those who are ill. Stephen wanted doctors to be kind, gentle and interested. Stephen tried hard to meaningfully converse with all his doctors; however, many doctors, Stephen would say, had 'cloth ears'.

He wanted bureaucracy destroyed so others did not have to go through its many little cruelties. Stephen loved the verse: 'Love is patient, love is kind. It does not envy, it does not boast, it is not proud. It is not rude, it is not self-seeking, it is not easily angered, and it keeps no record of wrongs. Love does not delight in evil but rejoices with the truth.'

Stephen wanted organisations to run with this verse in mind, not just on the wall plaque but in day-to-day practice.

Bureaucracy appears to be unavoidable in institutions that are supposed to care. Everyone blames the system, but who exactly is the system? The 'system' is created by faceless pen-pushers who do not utterly understand the needs of patients. The rigid rules they make do not have any flexibility nor the capacity to realise there is an exception to every rule.

Policies, procedures and rules are very necessary to provide structure in any organisation. If they do not leave room for common sense and interpretation according to the needs of the individual patient, however, they are nothing but oppressive and harmful. 'The system' has become a bureaucratic entity.

Here are some thoughts by Roger Montgomery, a member who helped start the band The Travelling Wheelchairies:

"For the first ten or so years of the seventeen years I worked there in full and part time positions as co-ordinator of the Woodwork Shop, I was mightily impressed and moved by the wonderful attitudes from the Staff and Management in treatments and caring. Dedicated volunteers also sought to make life easier for many courageous fragile young and older folk living permanently, by my book, in dire straits.

For those ten years it was glaringly obvious that the clients' welfare and happiness came first and foremost. It was a great place to work. I occasionally became involved in other activities, such as The Travelling Wheelchairies, working with a great Music Therapist. In one meeting with management, we got the go ahead and some funding for instruments and the like. That is all it took, one oral submission. Other musical instruments were supplied by a local music shop for naught.

Later, sadly, in my view, as the place became immersed and smothered by increasing governmental and bureaucratic wrangling, the standard of true and loving care waned. As costings increased and budgets decreased, all the un-caring coldness this engenders followed.

The result was a decrease in fun and play and caring, and in our case, budgets and complicated spreadsheets for the Workshop Clientele were being bruited about by outsiders saddled and bridled with governmental lack of compassion. As if life was not a big enough grind for our folk, without being frightened by some blundering governmental apparatchik pouring more uncertainty and fear upon their heads. Such a shame."

After Claire had left, we sat by Stephen's bed watching him breathe with the oxygen mask. He would periodically stop breathing and his blood oxygen level would go down, but after prompting him to take a few deep breaths, his oxygen would go up again. When he finally dropped off to sleep, he stopped breathing.

Alarmed, we called for help and minutes later, a doctor came and applied pressure underneath his brow. Stephen woke up and started breathing again. The doctor explained that the pressure upon pressing under his brow caused acute pain which had made him wake up. Stephen then settled down and went back to sleep for two hours, this time breathing evenly. We relaxed thinking he would get a good sleep and be better in the morning. Since his oxygen levels were now maintained, we left Stephen at 7:30 that night, thinking it was safe for us to go home.

I had just got to sleep when the phone rang. A male voice asked if I was Heather. I was alarmed, but was not expecting to hear these dreadful words:

"I am very sorry, your son Stephen passed away at 2:00 AM."

I screamed, handing the phone to Ray who was looking at me in horror. I could hardly believe what I had just heard. Ray spoke to the man for a minute or two and hung up. Then softly, he said to me, "We will get up to the hospital as soon as we get dressed."

On the way to the hospital, I was hyperventilating. I thought I was going to die too. Ray was driving too fast, and I said bleakly, "We don't have to speed towards a hospital any more for the first time in our lives." It felt like the longest drive ever.

Stevie had 'gone'.

When we arrived at the ward, we were greeted by several young nurses. They led us to Stephen's bed where he lay. I put my head on his chest as if to listen to him breathing and all I could feel was his cold skin on my face. I was overcome even more at his loss because I had not been with him when he died. We were both distraught that we had not stayed all night to monitor his oxygen levels.

Ray bent over and placed a kiss on his face. Stephen looked very peaceful. Despite the agony of grief, we were also relieved in a way that Stevie was no longer in pain.

The nurses all stood by, making cups of tea and asking if they could do anything. We just looked at Stephen and cried. After several hours just sitting beholding his face and trying to comprehend Stevie was no longer with us, we decided to go home, feeling distraught and lost over the loss of our brilliant loving son.

I bent over Stevie, and clutching his iPhone and watch, I whispered, believing somehow he could hear me, "I have your iPhone and your watch safe with me. Goodbye Stevie my beautiful boy."

It was 19 August, 2014, the end of a long and winding road.

We laid Stephen to rest on the morning of 27 August, 2014.

Eulogy by Geoff Usher delivered at Stephen's funeral

On behalf of Heather and Ray, I want to welcome you to this time of reflection on Steve's amazing life.

I first met Steve when he was 14 at my place of employment, which was a residential home with a school attached for disabled children. Stephen had arrived in Perth after several years of living in the USA, and I was a young orderly at the time.

I would arrive early to work to help Stephen out of bed to prepare for the day. My duties were to shower Stephen, take him to OT or physio and to and from school.

Our conversations were both lively and fun and at times intense and serious.

Our friendship grew and we had happy times together. We took Stephen to church in a bongo van that was kindly lent to us by a lady from church.

Stephen would often stay at our house on the weekends. He loved this and really enjoyed being part of our family. When Stephen's parents came back to visit from the USA, we enjoyed many outings together. My wife Fran visited Stephen weekly. He found her support invaluable.

When we moved away from the city, we kept in touch by phone with Stephen and found great encouragement by sharing our lives with each other.

Stephen chose to live his life with faith. He was the bravest guy I knew. I will always remember the day I baptised him in the Physio pool. He twitched, resulting in a fracture to his leg. Stephen's unrelenting courage and faith strengthened him.

We are here today mourning the absence of our wonderful son and friend. We are comforted knowing he fought the good fight and he is with Our Heavenly Father.

We will now have a few moments of reflection with a medley of some of Stephen's favourite songs: 'Soldier Boy', 'Here Comes the Sun', 'My Sweet Lord' and 'Let It Be'.

Eulogy by Claire delivered at Stephen's funeral

"Pssst, do you want a cushy job?" someone whispered to me during a coma-inducing lecture at nursing school. Without knowing details, I readily agreed. Little did I know the 'job' would turn into a twenty-year journey of transformative growth for me. Even though I turned up to be the 'carer', in time Stephen would become a full time 'God-sent' in my own life. Sometimes the greatest lessons in life can come from gifts in unusual wrappings; Stephen was one of those gifts for me. My life expanded because of him.

I first met Stephen when I was just 18 and we connected instantly. Awkward small talk before strangers become friends did not exist. I did not notice his physical disability. He was just him. Stephen irreverently poked fun at himself and his condition in a manner so disarmingly charming, that when one spent time with him his internal qualities shone. Despite the most difficult circumstances, he mocked his poor prognosis with authentic joy. Stephen was given cards in life from the Joker himself, spelling pain and suffering. Sure, he did not receive them passively without struggle, but embraced what he could not change graciously. Amidst those cards he still experienced times of intense happiness, fun and laughter. His skeleton was weak but his spirit strong. He lived by the principle: "If you don't like something, change it. If you cannot change it, change the way you think about it."

I recall we were getting him ready to go to the wedding of one of his carers. We dressed him in his best attire, but when we transferred him to his wheelchair, we noticed the power cord had been dislodged and consequently the battery was dead. This meant no mobility, so he had to stay home while we all went to the wedding. I will never forget how gracious he was. "You go and have a great time." He cheerily called as we set off, "Take lots of photos for me!" It would have been easy for him to become bitter by the unfairness of his situation. He rose above it.

In the time I knew Stephen, he was 3 feet and 1 inch tall (or perhaps I should say long, as it was measured lying down) which is the size of a boy. However, by definition, he was such a man. He never let me forget that inch if I were ever to describe his height to someone! Somehow, Stephen kept his head on when everything about his world was upside down. There was no natural progression in life though developmental milestones such as cars, marriage, careers, and children. Instead, he spent his life waiting – waiting for a bottle to be handed to him, waiting for medication to get out of pain, waiting for a cup of tea and waiting for an opportunity to help others. He had raw determination and grit. Despite incredible physical and emotional pain, he still reached out to others using tenderness and love. There is a lesson for all of us in that, including me.

Personal care for Stephen took time, so it allowed for a matrix of friendship to be built around us. He could clean his own teeth if you prepared the toothbrush and he could intermittently feed himself, but that's where independence started and ended. Stephen needed full assistance to shower and his meals had to be prepared by others. He did not have the luxury of getting up and making himself a ham sandwich if he felt like it. I was always struck by Heather and Ray's generosity in constantly opening their home to carers, day in and day out.

Despite his physical limitations and care requirements, Stephen's face was always expressive and his smile electric. Long lashes framed his round blue eyes set in a circular face and his voice often had notes of sheer happiness set within it when he was talking about subjects he loved. Conversations with Stephen were enlightening and stimulating, introducing me to a remarkable range of topics. We spent hours talking, and when I left for the day we continued by phone. Often, we laughed and said, lucky they do not charge per minute for local calls as if they did, we could not afford the bill. I repeatedly called him late in the night and after only one ring, I would be greeted with the ever reliable and sometimes sleep-induced croaky hello. As soon as I started to speak about the day's events, Stephen would always snap himself awake and focus his full attention on me.

Stephen was ALWAYS interested in whatever issue I had and available to help however he could. I was so blessed to have a 24-hour helpline with unbiased love and support. He was a true friend, and if I were doing something wrong, he would lovingly challenge me, not just agree with me for the sake of peace. That is the sign of a matured friend who only wanted the best for me. I could count on Stephen to be there when I needed him, not just in good times when things are going well but in bad times too. He never rejoiced when things went badly for me and he did not take me down a peg or two when things went well. I was loved by Stephen with no bounds, unconditionally and for no reason; he just loved me as I was. It was affection without limitations or conditions. It was unchanging no matter what happened between us. Stephen intrinsically knew the value of friendship. He shared his feelings with me and I with him. We were very real with one another. He made it a safe space to share. I did not know what I did to deserve that kind of friend. It was true companionship.

Stephen became a friend with a background completely different to anyone I have met yet he truly accepted me for who I was as a person. He would often quote the song 'I'll Stand By You' by The Pretenders. The lyrics include standing by someone through thick and thin and he particularly loved the line 'nothing you confess could make me love you less'. This made me feel safe. At the time when he repetitively quoted it, I was blasé about its practical application in my own life. I would tell him, "Yes, blah, blah, blah," – it's only now I see the full value of what he was trying to say and his genuine concern for me. I did not fully realise the significance of the line 'Let me see you through, because I've seen the dark side too.' Stephen indeed had seen the dark side of life with his trials and tribulations, yet he did not become bitter.

Friends are people whom you electively choose to be with, and Stephen and I chose each other. I was mesmerized by his supple brain which had such an analytical grasp, his width of interests, his humour and above all his ability to love.

A carpenter uses a saw and hammer to make furniture. A mechanic will use a spanner to fix a car. A stone mason will use a chisel. Stephen could not use physical tools. Instead, his tools were words, which he used to craft relationships of lasting value. He used the tool of words as an art. Stephen developed an inherent ability to help others with their psychological distress. He had the powerful intuition of knowing what to say for comfort. I watched him comfort the bereaved. He was able to communicate with people more than a mere exchange of information; he was able to do it in a way to 'connect' with them. He loved people not only for who they are, but for who they can become. His love had the power to make others aware of their potential and actualise it.

Stephen taught me the application of the Covey principles, things that are urgent are seldom important and things that are important are seldom urgent. He encouraged me to see what white noise was, and what was crucial in life and to live a life of simplicity before minimalism became fashionable.

Stephen's friendship was also practical in approach. He worried about my safety in case I broke down when driving and without stating the obvious he could not exactly grow a pair of legs and come and pick me up. In the days when mobile phones were the size and weight of a large house brick, he decided to purchase me one. Instantaneously I became the envy of my peers as mobile phones were only seen in films, they were not things for mere mortals to own. Everyone that saw it was amazed that little old me owned one. His motives were none other than altruistic, and he always wanted me to be safe. No wonder the symbol for love is hands joined in a heart shape – it is love in action.

Whenever he wrote in a birthday card, he would often include a little pen sketch done in great detail. It was made even more precious as it was drawn lying down and required physical effort of holding his leg stumps up to place the card on it so he could write on it. Stephen would say if he did not have this disease, he would have chosen to be an architect or music mixer. I think he would have been a combination of both.

I decided it was a good idea to show Stephen my world since he had told me so much about his, and one day we set off for Hope Valley where I grew up. He instantly became one of the family and whilst my brothers showed him their motorbikes, he did some burnouts in his wheelchair. We managed to lift his wheelchair into the back of a Volkswagen Kombi van and took him to the beach. Whilst lying on the trampoline, he was able to use a small plastic racket to hit a soft foam ball. We all chuckled as we affectionately called him the world's laziest tennis player.

At night, all the kids were talking and not sleeping. My mother yelled out in an Australian twang, "Get to sleep, you kids." We laughed about it for years afterwards. Stephen put a Bible verse up on my bedroom wall on a small innocuous looking card, which read: Love is patient. Love is kind... (1 Corinthians 13, v 4-8), as he never wanted me to forget it. Ironically, it could be re-read as Stephen was patient, Stephen was kind, etc.

We had such fun together with a steady flow of satirical commentary about how society worked. He intuitively knew how to make me laugh and see the funny side of situations, no matter how dire his circumstances. One of Stephens's gifts was the accurate observation and assessment of human behaviour and to see through people's motives. Stephen had an innate ability to cut through surface issues. When I discussed anyone else's actions with him, he was able to explore the details with me, then expose motives that were inconspicuous to me. He was always right and helped me safely navigate many tricky situations.

I have the fondest memories of Stephen's hugs. He would hug you with his bent arm which would stick into your back. He was the only person who could stretch out his arm to hug you, but his hand would be pointing in the opposite direction.

In times when Stephen's spine was able to tolerate sitting longer, I would fill my passenger seat with cushions, then lift him into the car and take him driving. I obviously operated the pedals and from the passenger seat he steered with his right arm. The police never pulled us over, but any fine incurred was worth it. The smile on Stephen's face was priceless. He steered confidently and with ease like a seasoned pro and navigated his way easily across dual carriage ways. I was worried we were going to crash; however, he reassured me he had already steered across America several times and was not planning to crash anytime soon. Years later as his spine deteriorated and he was no longer able to sit up, technology had improved so I would Skype him by mounting my iPad on the dashboard. It was a great way to bring my world to him.

When Stephen's parents holidayed overseas, they asked me to stay with Stephen. He and I lived in bliss. We ate junk food, watched loads of cable TV, and played loud music. We rebelled against conventional regimes and did not keep a proper day/night routine. We had simple fun and it was glorious.

Stephen taught me the true meaning of what is universally known as the Golden Rule – treat others as you would like to be treated. Everything in life is much easier and more joyful if you follow this. Stephen taught me to be practical and look for what the patient needed, not how the patient could be fit in a rigid health system. This lesson was unbelievably valuable and changed my outlook as a nurse.

Multiple support pillows needed careful precise placement under Stephen to ensure fractures did not follow. Making his bed would take several minutes and then it would take a long time to get him comfortable. If things were not in the exact position, it could cause him discomfort. It taught me not just about the placement of pillows, but to make the patient feel psychologically safe enough to ask for what they needed.

I often wondered where Stephen got his strength from. He was always self-deprecating and took no credit for having faith. He humbly said others had helped him along the way in his journey and for this he was grateful. He simply believed all things work together for the good. Despite his future being overshadowed by physical disability, he committed to a rich interior life.

He discovered the best use of his life was love, the best expression of love was time and the best time to love was NOW and in every breath he took. Love helped him push through every challenge. Regardless of Stephen's disability, he had a reason and purpose to live and a meaningful contribution to make to the world. Life with a chronic illness has a diversely coloured bouquet of fears, joys, sorrows, pains, choices and opportunities. Stephen reviewed and reordered his life's priorities; his priorities were relationships and to support people. He desperately wished to improve communication with healthcare professionals and controlling his pain better, but sadly this was not always achievable. At times, bureaucrats considered Stephen was being difficult; the reality is, he was being human.

One night after a lengthy phone conversation, I crawled into bed and slept soundly. The next morning there were pages and pages of xxxxxx, all in, over 90 texts each containing the same message xxx xxx xxx xxx xxx. It was 14 Aug, 2014, 4:50 PM. I laughed heartily and thought how much I treasured and valued my special friendship with Stephen. Every 'x' made my heart sing, but it was the message that came almost at the very bottom that touched me the most: 'God bless and love you, Claire'. At the time I had no idea this was the last message I would ever receive from him.

The following day, Stephen became unwell and was taken to hospital in an ambulance. Late that night, my deep sleep was interrupted by the melodious ring of the iPhone. It was Stephen. His voice was clear and lucid. "I'm at the hospital but I'm home," he announced proudly.

I was delighted to hear his robustness. His previous breathlessness had disappeared, and he sounded happy and excited. "What do you mean you are home?" I retorted. "You are in hospital."

"No, no, I'm at the hospital, but I'm home," he responded. "I know I'm home."

"You sound like you are confused to me, just go to sleep. I will talk to you tomorrow," I replied. I hung up delighted to hear his voice so strong and I had full faith and confidence my boy was better. I pulled the covers back up and slept intoxicated with contentment. My boy was on the mend.

At 4:30 AM, the shrill sound of the phone ringing ferociously pierced the pre-dawn cool air again. Earlier the phone had sounded melodious, this time it sounded menacing. I sat bolt upright with fear and trepidation. Ray told me Stephen was gone. I was stunned.

Complete shock, numbness and a sense of implausibility prevailed. This could not be real.

Stephen's faith was strong, and he faced death courageously. Some of us are alarmed and frightened of death, but not him. Several months before he died, he sent a random text message to say how beautiful heaven was, that it will be 'easy, peaceful and beautiful'. In my final conversation with Stephen, he did say he was 'home'. I now appreciate the significance of the last text message he sent me and believe he had one leg already in the door of heaven when I spoke to him for the last time.

His life was bathed in bureaucracy. When Stephen was born, Ray rang the hospital and they would not tell him whether Heather had given birth or not. How could we not laugh, when 54 years of dealing with health rules and regulations concluded in the grand finale of collecting Stephen's ashes. When signing the paperwork to release his ashes, Ray's signature looked ever so marginally different. We were not given permission to take Stephen's ashes with us despite our own copious ID documents. "We are unable to give you his ashes," we were told in the same curt tone that had informed Ray that he was unable to find out if he was a father or not, all those years earlier. Bureaucracy had come full circle: from birth to death, and without a single day's sleep in between.

Stephen lived more in his life than most, despite not being able to walk since the age of eight, not able to sit up by himself since age 14, and being bed bound for the last 20 years of his life, apart from going to the toilet for which he also had to lie down. Most use just their eyes to see, but Stephen used a combination of heart, brain, and eyes to see. He saw past external situations and lived a more rounded life than many able-bodied people. Because of Stephen, my heart is no longer in the lovely shape you have seen on greeting cards on Valentine's Day. It has been stretched beyond recognition then broken with his passing, yet it has been glued back together stronger than it was before I met him. The journey I have gone through with him has changed my heart's landscape irreversibly, for the better.

Stephen, my friend, your courage in adversity, empathy for others and ability to combine intelligence and heart were your greatest gifts.

Thank you for teaching me how to have a happy life through your formula or the 3 F's:

Faith: To have an attitude of trust that everything will be okay, no matter what the current circumstances are.

Friendships: These are key to helping you survive any challenge.

And most of all,

Fun: You taught me to see humour in any situation and humour is the best tool to navigate life. I will remember your lessons forever.

Visiting hours are now over, but your legacy lives on. RIP Stephen, until we meet again.

Eulogy by Lester Farnam delivered at Stephen's funeral

Stephen, my friend, I miss your famous greeting: that infinite smile, a mischievous playfulness, always an engaging long firm handshake, even at the risk of personal injury to your precious bones.

I do find comfort though, listening to you now, whispering those profound and melodious words of wisdom: "Let it be."

I first met you, Stephen, sometime in the early eighties, in the previous century. You could always tell me the exact year, month, and perhaps in jest, even the day; so sharp was your mind.

My hobby at the time was exposing institutions for what they are: non places of the heart. I wanted to get into a particular organisation to take photos. Funny, because you wanted to get out!

I volunteered as photographer tutoring in composition, exposure, and developing and printing; but it was you who soon captured my imagination, with your insatiable curiosity, indefatigable energy, and natural wit. One might say we shared a similar sensibility.

The rapport was immediate, and thus began a lifelong friendship. We soon discovered that our mutual interests extended to multitrack recording. We eagerly collaborated in mixing party tapes, set about creating serenades for unsuspecting females; we just enjoyed the thing in itself: That sheer delight in bringing together two or more bits of audio, and thereby enhancing any musical effect.

You were a virtual student of George Martin, the producer and audio engineer for the Beatles. Under your tutelage, I mastered many recording techniques including an understanding of peak level monitoring; signal to noise ratio; expanding dynamic range with DBX. Electronic circuitry compared to Dolby noise suppression systems; and the realization that there are subtle differences between ferrous oxide chrome and metal-based tapes. All this I can remember from our days as amateur technicians.

Mate! You had the most prodigious intellect! Your mum recently told me that you have an IQ of 180, a genius. She also told me you were ranked number one in your matriculation score for a university in the United States of America. You were accepted for entry, but for reasons known to you, you failed to follow through. You never mentioned it to me, being so humble I suppose.

I love to travel and have a need to go and see the world for myself. I am an empiricist. Your world was more inner, abstract, and representational, rather than experiential. Your explorations revolved around your beloved Apple Mac. You would forever subject me to images on your huge twenty-seven-inch computer display.

Your incessant creativity was aroused in virtual space: mostly in science and mathematics. Little excited you more than enthusiastically sharing your discoveries with others. Your many interests included fascinations with such notions as: Symmetry; Colour; Optics; Mandelbrot set theory (or Fractals) and Boolean Geometry - not content at merely using a computer - you had to also understand the historical development of computing itself.

You were seldom happier than when adventuring into the elegant equations of mathematical logic, finding joy in discovering aspects of the microcosm (Humanity); becoming excited with explorations of the macrocosm (The Universe); being in touch with beauty itself was what turned you on. Actually, you never really switched off.

It would be an understatement to say you were intense. Your overactive mind was always overflowing with energy. Your only downtime, it seemed to me, is when you were comfortably numbed by sleep! I'll share a secret with you. At times I felt overwhelmed in your presence, experiencing a need to escape and a strong urge to flee. Taking refuge into my relatively much slower paced, simpler existence was for me, a defence mechanism.

I found you to be strong willed yet also gracious. Except on one occasion, whilst I was under contract to supply services to you, I was sacked for insubordination! Mate, do you remember that? Come to think of it, I rushed away so quickly, I can't recall whether or not you paid me! I'll send you the invoice sometime.

For a while now, you have confined yourself to bed. I remember when you first declined to come out with me. Before that occurrence, we sometimes went out together, usually to visit friends, go to a party, attend a concert, or shop for Apple, Yamaha, or TDK products. It isn't that you are by nature a private person; going out merely hurt too much.

On one occasion, following a short trip in my 4WD, those sore bones of yours troubled you for weeks afterwards. However, the avoidance of activity does not guarantee any cessation of pain. Most of your life you have been faced with a stark choice: that between pain-induced activity and pain-induced inactivity. Unsurprisingly, you prefer it now, if people come to you, and visits are always received with the greatest of pleasure.

Perhaps there is no greater example of your love and appreciation of beauty, than your deep passion for music.

Bones may be brittle, but they are enthused with soul. You have such sensitivity for music, both in the technical and aesthetic sense. Over time, you have introduced me to much good song and instrumentation.

Idiosyncratically, you tend to present only parts of the whole, the bits that stand apart, in your mind, from the totality. You have the proverbial ear for the superlative, and you are keen in subjecting me, and others, analytically, to the rewind and fast-forward function, ad infinitum. I am always surprised you do not wear out your tape heads more often.

No easy listening! Why, for example, are we never, as when I am with my normal friends, permitted to simply play the piece through?

It was you who introduced me to this music that we can hear now: Beethoven's Fifth piano concerto in E flat major. You have a particular interest, and I'll never forget it, at the interface between the ascending chord progression, at the end of the adagio un poco mosso of the second movement leading perfectly into the rondo allegro at the beginning of the third movement.

My memory behaves like the properties of iron in the ferromagnetism on the tape itself. That is to say, you successfully etched a groove in my brain, due to your repetitive demonstrations.

You played the piano, at least until the bones in your hands began to react adversely to pressure from the keyboard. Latterly, you have found the air piano more conducive, and more forgiving, and I might add, it sounds better too!

Before meeting you, I had never the pleasure of knowing a Beatle maniac. Not content with the mere appreciation of lyrics or melody, you can happily rattle off: dates; venues; production data; the line-up, including any session musicians; any orchestral instruments that have been employed; whether it was take one, take two, take three, or whichever take used for the single or album release - and being the quintessential muso yourself - elucidate to me, abstractions such as: key signature, octave changes, and pitch variation employed in any piece.

As I alluded to above, it was never easy listening with you. Stephen, you do not want for much, as your life is rich enough already. Like your good mate John Lennon, all you need is love, and your wish is to be loved in return.

Despite your different abilities, you do not ask for much. Your only requirement is to be able to live as normal a life as you can. Your want, is to maintain personal control over your life, and to be, as free of pain, as is chemically possible. Unfortunately, these outcomes seldom eventuate, yet characteristically, you always soldier on.

Recall you, cheery as ever; being admitted to hospital to have your legs cut off. The pain in your legs had got so bad. Mate, when faced with adversity, you are peerless. Who amongst us gathered here today, could have the fortitude to undertake a double amputation, just to make one's day a little more bearable?

Upping an already maxed out prescription of painkillers would not be an option, as the tolerance levels of the body can only adapt to so much.

Oh! What unimaginable suffering. I don't even want to think about it. In your case Stephen, suffering is tempered with just the right balance of strength. Imagine every day having to find the resources to face the difficulties that a life of dependency entails, not just of the physical kind either:

Repeatedly having to hold out against the medical fraternity; fend off the legal fraternity; and stand up to the caring fraternity - all of whom have vested interests of their own –

Stephen, you have held up under enormous pressure. I would say, much of your potency arises, not only due to a steely resolve, but from a deep and personal, real, and lively spirituality. At least once, you have benefitted from some good luck, as you inherited one tower, and one pillar of strength: Two of the most loving, caring, generous and devoted beings. Together, they have provided you with the perfect support system, and they continue to watch over you today, Mother Heather, and Father Ray.

So too, throughout your life, you have gained resilience from the multitude of hearts whom you have touched, with your heartfelt love; and the countless minds, who have been forever altered by your presence, some, of the many of whom, stand here with you now, as a testament to the love you have shown them.

Finally, I beseech you to hold onto this image for a while: Stephen, you were born from a soothing amniotic fluid. In this photograph,

I present you with here, you are enjoying a momentary refuge from the pressure and from the pain that gravity exerts upon your fragile skeletal musculature. Weightlessness.

It is no wonder that you fantasised about being in space. If there may come a time from whence, I might feel no pain - in my case, emotional pain - I would feel I was, indeed, in heaven. Steve, I bet you are rather surprised, to hear me utter that? Perhaps you have caught me in a moment of vulnerability?

It is with some solace, in my mind at least, that with your passing, all the incessant pain, which was destined to be your burden, and which, over a lifetime, you had to endure, has finally departed your body, and has left you free.

"Free at last" (words borrowed from Martin Luther King Jr.) "Free as a Bird," (John Lennon's final Beatle song.)

Stephen, my old mate. My most enduring friend in Perth.

Visiting Hours are now over, I'm afraid.

I love you, always have; always will.

Your friend, Lester.

PART 6: TRIBUTES TO STEPHEN

Nic, friend

I first met Stephen on 18th August 2006. I well remember the warm welcome I received when Heather opened the door to let this stranger into the home.

Being ushered into Stephen's room, I was given the same warm friendly welcome. This initial encounter turned my visitor status into a friendship status. In the next eight years of frequent and infrequent visits, this warmth of welcome never varied.

Stephen had a wonderful engaging way about him. He was a great conversationalist. He shared freely on any topic be it music, his first love, maths, science, and geography. He was also interested to tap into my story line. He had a remarkable ability to identify fully with those visiting him.

As time went on, he became mesmerised by the electronic media. This provided even more stimulation and interests. With Stephen there were never moments of awkward silence because Steve loved to make the most of the time.

He had to embrace the many different carers assigned to him over many years. Nearly all carers provided more stimuli because many came from other countries and cultures. The encounters were rich but also sad because most were short term carers. I never heard Steve complain but he did feel the pain of severed friendships.

Steve climbed a mountain that most of us are not required to negotiate, and he did it over such a long period of time. He remained optimistic while traversing the valleys, plateaus as well as the sharp ridges of pain and frustration. What gave the most pain were the moments when professionalism got in the way of hearing his cry for understanding.

In the whole journey of life, you indicated that you were sustained from within by the person, who said,

“I will never leave you nor forsake you.”

You acknowledge the Lord Jesus as your Saviour who kept you in faith as you travelled this difficult and complex journey.

Steve, you have been and are a wonderful inspiration and I thank you and your parents for allowing me the privilege to enter into a brief period of your journey. Now that the journey is complete the Lord will renew your total person. We wait to share that experience with you.

From your grateful friend Nic, whom you enriched and inspired with your person.

Brad, carer, friend

I came to know Steve around 1996.He was living in Brentwood when I became one of his carers. His mother was staying with him.

We were the same age, and had a lot in common, mostly music from the 60s and 70s, English pop bands, rock bands and English humour. In free time we spent hours listening and watching our era’s entertainment on TV.

Steve lived on his bed and most days used his computer. I listened while he taught me all about Apple computers. Just to be annoying I said

“I liked Bill Gates and IBM.”

We reminisced about our childhood and Steve’s life growing up in America. He had been around the world with his parents. I learned a lot about his life.

Steve had a lot of insight living with constant pain and the health system. It was a long and intense life of pain he had lived. There was no cure for his disease and in the end most pain treatments were nowhere near what he needed.

Comedy was a temporary escape and we had plenty of laughs. Steve was a good sport when I played practical jokes on him. He loved music especially the Beatles, and Abby Road music studio. He was greatly interested in sound engineering. He knew everything about the Beatles and the way they produced all their records.

It was with Steve I soon learned the difficulty of severe suffering with no cure in sight. His problem with chronic pain and navigating through the health system was complexed and had many twists and turns. Pain specialists and many visits to hospital and doctors' surgeries, could not bring his pain to a place where he could live comfortably in his own skin.

To endure through this, Steve and his family had to go into endless cycles with doctors and pain medication, making it worse. The strongest medicines only became less affective after time. It seemed after many trials his life was going to be in continuous pain until he died in 2014.

It was just that. No matter of trying and many medical interventions, his bones and brain could find little relief.

It was a struggle of torment and sweat most days for Steve, which could leave all people involved frustrated.

Being too sore to get himself his medicine, he relied on the people who looked after him for help. By law carers where not allowed to do this, which led to many troubles and difficulties in his daily life.

Steve's parents went through all this suffering and troubles with him, and they too went through all the strain till the last. I take my hat off to all of those to have to live his type of life.

When people have a lifetime of extreme medical conditions the medical need is great, but it was also a huge sorrow. There were many doctors and arguments, and a merry go round trying to solve the pain problem which never stopped.

There are many illnesses that I wish could be cured and pain is one of the biggest. It drains you all day long, making easy things hard to do. In his own way Steve was quite stoic because long suffering was hard to endure. It took so much a strong state of mind to endure what Stephen went through.

I will remember him as a good friend, unique and a little Aussie battler. One of life's stories that needs to be told.

Laura, carer, friend

Stephen was such a totally unique amazing individual, he had so many stories to tell of happy times and tougher times also but through every challenge he has faced he never lost his persona of positivity! I will always cherish the time I worked for you guys and the times we've spent together.

Conor, carer, friend

I had the pleasure of working with Stephen in 2011–2012 whilst on a working holiday visa in Australia after finishing university back home in Ireland. I can recall meeting Stephen for the first time in March 2011 in his home in Kardinya that he shared with his wonderful parents, Heather, and Ray.

I was struck by Stephen's positive, friendly, and outgoing demeanour despite his severe physical disabilities. There was rarely a dull moment due to Stephen's dry wit and sense of humour. For me working, Stephen brought new experiences such as getting to listen to The Beatles back catalogue and watching Aussie comedies like Kath and Kim. I recall Stephen's infectious cackle! Stephen was a great storyteller. He loved talking about his time living in America and his travels in Europe in particular driving around London looking for the Abbey Road pedestrian crossing! Even thought he was restricted in his physical abilities; this did not stop Stephen from maintaining friendships through Skype and accessing the world through the medium of Google Earth.

Stephen could always show up my technophobic side with his tech savvy ways. Some of my favourite memories with Stephen are so simple. For me, the fondest memories were afternoons sitting outside in the garden catching some rays of sunshine and petting the family pets, Peggy Sue, and Ruby Jean. We would sit and listen to music and put the world to rights.

Stephen was so open-minded and worldly. He loved learning new things – mimicking one another's accent comes to mind. Stephen would exclaim through laughter that I sounded so 'ocker Aussie' in my attempts!

In my time working with Stephen, I got to know Heather and Ray and his dear friend Claire. A great perk at Kardinya was Heather's delicious home cooked food. Heather and Ray welcomed carers into their home and were so caring and supportive.

I enjoyed meeting Heather and Ray for a Guinness in Dublin in 2015. I stopped working with Stephen in May 2012 and have fond memories in the leaving party that the Simpsons threw for me. A Great laugh was had. I kept in touch with Stephen on Facebook until his sad passing.

I was honoured to know Stephen and I will never forget the laughs we had and the fond memories of my time in Australia.

Linda, carer, friend

It was the year 1995 in October, I first met Steve when he was living on his own and he was moving back into his parent's house. Heather and I were packing up his things. We did a few trips to and from the houses. I remember there were shelves full of video tapes.

I had spoken to Steve on the phone before starting work. I really didn't know what to expect only that he sounded really nice. I only knew his disease was brittle bones! So, when I first met him face to face, I was a little shocked by how deformed his arms were and how little he looked! But he had a beautiful smile and a gentle kind voice so that made me feel extremely comfortable!

Steve spent most of the time in bed, so I helped Heather pack boxes! I remember there were shelves full of videos tapes! Lol

When Steve was ready to get up for his shower, I was very nervous as I had to lift him as gently as I could on to the shower chair It all went well, and I stayed working for Steve for over 2 years. I started work 2 days a week, and increased working 4 days being Friday, Saturday, Sunday, and Monday.

I would stay over most weekends! It was really great because Steve then could get up for his shower when he felt pain free! Sometimes it would take till 5PM to feel ok.

Friday nights Heather would have a boot scooting class! Steve would then play his music. He had a great sound system, and he would crank the music up. If he was in his wheelchair, we would be dancing around the lounge room. It was so much fun.

Most days after Steve had his shower, we would go for a walk, down to the park if we only had a short amount of time. Otherwise, we would go walking around the suburbs. Steve loved looking at the architecture. We would be gone for hours, and always took Stephen's dog Lilly with us.

I remember one day I had to drive Steve to the Hospital. He was sitting in the passenger seat as we were driving along the freeway. He asked if he could steer the car. I said "for sure" so he took the wheel with his stronger right arm while I pretended to be looking in the mirror with my hands in the air. We were looking at the drivers going in the opposite direction observing us with shock and wonder. It made us laugh. Steve had a great sense of humour.

Steve's 40th birthday was a super day because Heather had all her fabulous friends over for a boot scooting party. Steve was in his wheelchair dancing away. Do you remember that, Heather?

You must miss him so much. He was an amazing person.

Thanks so much for your patience, Heather.

Look after yourselves.

Lots of love

Michael, carer, friend

Stephen and I shared a common interest in music. We had some great times together. I remember one memorable time when we ran our own version of Live Aid using videos recorded by those living together and then ran the full 24 hours using a donated large screen TV. Stephen was instrumental in putting together the audio visuals. On the day Stephen had a great time, zooming around in his wheelchair on the dance floor! Happy memories, Stephen.

Rico

Steve would come to my workshop regularly and we would listen to the Beatles and talk about the group Think Pink by the Fabulous Poodles which was a spoof on the Beatles music. It always was a pleasure having him around and to be able to help him with his mobility and comfort needs which were many.

I am so pleased that he made a commitment to Christ and now is in The Lord's care I have many wonderful memories of Steve which will always be with me.

Jodie, friend

Stephen was an amazing person and a wise old soul. I used to look forward to our weekly catch ups which were deep and meaningful.

Stephen loved his Apple computer and when this was not working, it limited his freedom of speech, and ability to advocate for himself and other people with disabilities.

He oozed passion and equality for all. He imparted wisdom and knowledge with all that he came into contact with. Our time was short, but I am blessed and thankful our paths crossed. You are forever in my heat Stephen and may you soar to new heights.

Yotam, carer

When you go into the garden, you will see a lot of plants. There will be one flower the brightest colour that stands out amongst the garden that is how Stephen was.

Chris, friend, carer

I first met Stephen in December 2011. I was invited in by a carer already attending to Stephen. When I entered Stephen's room, and seeing him, my countenance changed from being relaxed to having mixed feelings of compassion, and anxiety. Overcome, I dashed out of his bedroom to the bathroom.

I found myself shedding tears but quickly I said a prayer for Stephen as I had not seen a person in such a condition before in my life. After a few moments I went back to Stephen's room and apologised for the unkind gesture, but Stephen accepted my apology and reassured me that he understood my reaction.

Stephen explained to me his condition, his medicines and how to take care of him to which I quickly found myself having feelings of being calm and accepted by him. My journey with Stephen had begun. I recall many precious moments with Stephen. We shared plenty of jokes and laughter.

In between, we had many arguments about fixing his numerous pillows needed for supporting each leg. His hip had become frozen at 30 degrees due to multiple fractures and the way it healed. His left arm required support and underneath his neck required a several towels strategically placed for support. It was difficult to find the most comfortable position.

He taught me a lot about the word of God and the bible. Mostly he taught me what the bible stood for when it came to marriage. I remember one day after looking at the topic we decided to ask Google what if Google thought marriage was good and Google said "no" we laughed together.

I remember the time Stephen was admitted into hospital. I was at home when I received a call from Stephen. He asked me if I would come and stay with him. When I arrived, Stephen was sleeping. When he woke up after midnight the room was dark. Stephen did not recognise me until the nurse told him that Chris was here. "Chris my brother," he said with such joy and his beautiful big smile. He grabbed my hand, shaking it vigorously, so that I was worried he would break a bone.

I spent the night on the floor. He wanted to pay me, but I told him that was not necessary. He was always mindful of not taking advantage of other people.

I left in the morning feeling sad to leave him in the hospital, but I had to attend a lecture at the university.

Stephen shared his life with me. I felt privileged which was special to me because he opened up the intimacy of his life. He told me how much he loved two girls in his life he fell deeply in love with.

The last time I saw Stephen was on a Thursday when I was asked to take him to the hospital for a bone scan. I put him in the van and had problems doing up the straps to secure him. I was mindful of being careful of his bones.

At the hospital, the nurses and the doctors did not know how to transfer him from the wheelchair because of the possibility of breaking his bones so I lifted him in my arms onto the hospital bed. After the bone scan, I took him back home. A few days later I got the unfortunate news that Stephen had sadly left this world.

Peter, carer

Stephen came to our disability house with much apprehension. There was nothing to fear. He settled in the house with ease, and he was not going to fall apart with just looking at him which was a relief to all the carers.

I would like to acknowledge Stephen's exceptional supportive mother and father Heather and Ray and dear friend Claire of which Stephen always spoke so highly of. Stephen's attitude to life was moulded by these wonderful people in his life.

Stephen had a lovely disposition, polite easy-going nature, and a fantastic sense of humour with many interests. He loved music, general knowledge, and his love of anything Apple although in regard to the latter, much to his frustration. Stephen could get frustrated and angry at times but to Stephen's credit he would always apologise. As carer it is a trait we do not always experience.

One day Stephen called out,

"Peter, would you get a bit of paper and write down a password for me?"

Stephen was always forgetting his passwords. So, we set about creating a password with all the secrecy of a Freemasons ritual. Half a page later and with numinous scratching, I had to say to Stephen,

"Steve you are making this too complicated."

Very fond memories of sitting with Stephen at night after all the other residents were in bed this was Stephen's time listening to music discussing many topics, music, planes, laughing at comedy shows, is there a God.

Stephen always had something he had discovered on the internet to show me and discuss.

Being a carer for many years Stephen stands out as a most memorable guy. I always looked forward to coming on shift to see Stephen.

Repinda, carer

Who could not forget Stephen? His personality was huge, and he cared for others.

Charmaine, friend

I met Stephen for the first time on skype. My husband Chris was his carer. They became close friends and considered each other brothers. Chris and I were only dating at the time. As brothers I am certain they had many conversations about me before I finally got to meet Stephen.

Stephen shared with me his love for music by telling me about his favourite bands and playing their songs for me.

Each time Chris was with Stephen, I would be sure to receive a call from the brothers. Music was not Stephen's only passion. He was a dedicated Christian who always had a story or verse to share. I found this challenging because I was going through hard times, but he had been through worse and still managed to maintain his relationship with God, so much so that he would convey a quote from the bible for every problem known to man.

This renewed my love for God, and I began to understand how special Stephen was. At first sight, I was overcome by feelings of sorrow for his condition, but once I got to know him, I realised, he was full of knowledge and life.

My husband and I were in a long-distance relationship when we were dating, and communication was the lifeline of our love. I was in Zambia while he was in Australia and it was challenging to link our different time zones in a way that we could spend enough time talking without clashing with each other's schedules.

Chris and I had made it a point in our relationship to never go a day without communicating. This particular day I did not hear from Chris. Typically, I began to imagine all sorts of things that could have happened to him. It was not like him to behave this way. When he finally called and I realised he was ok, I got so angry with him and didn't want to talk.

I then got a call probably About 30 minutes later from a number I did not recognise. "Hi Charmaine, this is Steve" he said. I was happy to hear his voice but wondered why he was calling me. Usually, Chris would call first via skype, and then introduce Stephen to our conversation.

He told me he knew that I was upset with Chris and was not speaking to him that day. As a brother would, he vouched for Chris, and assured me that Chris was a good man and would never do anything to jeopardise our relationship. Stephen went further and began to speak about the Gospel of John from the Holy Bible, 1 John 4:7-21. It speaks of love and faith.

After a good bible session and lecture on love and forgiveness, he asked if I would like to speak with Chris. How could I say no? The man just quoted the bible and set my head back on track. I agreed to speak with Chris and the rest is history.

Stephen was a peacemaker who wanted people around him to genuinely be happy. He found joy in seeing others happy.

Epilogue

After the Angels came down and guided Stephen's spirit up to heaven, Peggy Sue, our dog, ran around the house barking at nothing and nobody for three days. Ruby Jean, Stephen's faithful cat, lay down on the floor for hours where his bed used to be.

The loss of our dear Stevie rendered feelings of helplessness and deep pain. I felt as if I was chocking. I could not imagine our life without him. Claire and our close friends rallied around us, helping with funeral arrangements.

Claire always asked me the whole time while writing this book, "How did you not go mad with all that pain?" I told her I always had hope things would get better and besides hope, love for my son gave me strength to press on.

Stephen was so well loved by his friends, carers, and family. He encountered many people from different walks of life and different backgrounds. They all expressed the same admiration about his character.

Because of his painful disability and the battles with bureaucracy, Stephen developed wisdom beyond his years and was a gift in the lives of many. He listened to them, helped, and supported them. Stephen took on the role of carer for others, in such a way, it was transformative for them. The patient became the healer.

We three saw the world together. We brought joy to one another whether Stephen was with us, or by the Internet Café and Skype, whenever we were travelling, and when he was bedridden. He lived more in his life on earth than most people, even with his disability.

Stephen saw the wheel of life through his heart. He never suffered from self-pity. Despite his own challenges, he was able to care for the wellbeing of others unselfishly and genuinely. He was the ideal gentleman.

Although Stephen's skeleton was fragile and his bones misshapen, it did not stop us from taking him all over the world until his mid-twenties. Stephen was academically and musically gifted, with a great sense of humour that carried him through hard times. I am comforted by remembering his infectious laughter, where he would hold onto his ribs to prevent them from breaking when he laughed. Also, two words he used were so witty. Whenever he won an argument, and his rival was stuck for words, Stephen would say "Shattered" or "Jolted," to them, ending the disagreement, always made me laugh.

I have noted that a sense of humour, and courage, are distinguishing qualities of many with a disability.

Despite multiple fractures, Stephen showed great fortitude. Paradoxically his bones were weak, but his spirit had a steely resolve stronger than titanium. His heart was big and his courage admirable. In spite of his own disability, he reached out to many with care and friendship. Because of his own dilemma, it was apparent to me that he had an intrinsic ability to understand the difficulties of others and to reach out to them with compassion.

Stephen died peacefully on 19th August, 2014, aged 54, and has left an enduring legacy of admiration for us and his many friends.

Acknowledgments

I want to thank you, Ray, my husband, for your love and support and for always taking good care of me, in good days and bad days, for over 60 years.

Thank you to my brother Tom for filling in the gaps when writing about me as a little girl.

Thank you to my dear friend Claire for dedicating your time in helping me write my book. I am grateful for the fun we had together. I look back and think about us as a great team. Your input, as Stephen's carer and true friend, has been invaluable.

Thank you, Linda, Leon, and Claire for dedicating your time in building the monitor-holder that hung from Stephen's lifting hoist, a brilliant achievement greatly adding to his ease and comfort, and allowing him countless hours of pleasure, with the image directly in front of him rather than off to one side.

Grateful recognition goes to Megan Brown for her technical help and support throughout the time it took me to write my story.

Thank you to each and every one of Stephen's Carers, genuinely loving human beings, helping me too, above and beyond their duties. You are my heroes.

About The Author

Heather Simpson was born in Fremantle, Western Australia, in 1940. She was born with a painful brittle bone disease called Osteogenesis Imperfecta.

She married Raymond Simpson and had a son, Stephen, born with the same bone disease.

The three moved to Port Hedland, Western Australia, and from there emigrated to Wyoming, USA, in the late '60s in hopes of finding a cure for their son's disease. She attended Wyoming College and later Huntsville University in Alabama.

They travelled all over America. After 20 years and a downturn in the economy, they moved back to Perth, Western Australia, where she obtained work as a word processor in a major law firm.

This is her first book, based on their travels and their son's bone disorder. She describes how they navigated through life with humour, music and faith, with the hope of helping others dealing with this debilitating bone condition.

www.ingramcontent.com/pod-product-compliance
Ingram Content Group UK Ltd.
Pitfield, Milton Keynes, MK11 3LW, UK
UKHW062312290726
14090UKWH00018B/1021